Shine

The Silver Lining of Living with Cancer
is God's Love, the Greatest Gift of All.

Laura Dahl

ISBN 978-0-9833848-9-2
Published by
Susan the Scribe, Inc.
Ponte Vedra Beach, FL 32082
www.susanthescribe.vpweb.com
Graphic Design by
Trish Diggins
www.trishdiggins.com

For Steve, Rachel, Benjamin, Katherine, and Aaron
- the great loves of my soul.

To Susan Brandenburg,

My teacher, my dear friend, my light.

Thank you so much for showing how to do this book and Who it's all about.

You are such a great blessing and I consider myself lucky to have met you and have you help me.

Laura Dahl

prologue

In February of 2009, at 39 years old, I was diagnosed with Stage 4 Breast Cancer, which has since metastasized to my brain. I started writing this book a couple of years ago, realizing that I really wanted a written story about my cancer journey for my husband and our four children. With those "practice" years under my belt, God has been prodding me recently to finish up. I don't think I was ready to take the project on and still had too much yet to experience in my cancer journey. I don't know if this new enthusiasm is a message, but I feel like the time is now. I am supposed to finish what I started because the message needs to get out.

I have especially wanted to focus on how I got through the whole mess. In the beginning, the news that you've got cancer is overwhelming to say the least. As you read through my story, you will understand how God has gotten me through. God has plans for us. A neighbor once told me if you want to make God laugh, tell Him your plans. I think he was right on the target!

God is the center of my universe and I am so thankful we

have a relationship where He hears my prayers and supports my life. In fact, I believe He physically supports me! Without Him, my life would have been over long ago. It was in 2003, long before cancer, that I attended my first Cursillo and it changed my life. A Cursillo is a three day weekend, all men or all women, and centers on one's spirituality. It means "short course in Christianity" and can be that for some, but for me, it was major. From the website champaigncursillo.com:

> *A Cursillo weekend begins on a Thursday evening and ends on Sunday night. During the three days the participants listen to the Gospel message given in fifteen short talks. Five talks are given by clergy that center on Grace, the gift of God to all persons. The other ten are given by lay persons that have made a Cursillo. The talks deal with Christian study, action, leadership, living a life in relationship with God, the role of the layperson in the church and similar reflections on situations encountered in daily living. The talks build on each other.*

Truly knowing Jesus for the first time actually prepared me for what was to come. After going to Cursillo, I began praying to God every day that if anything bad was to happen to anyone in my family – anything life-threatening like a car accident, sickness, whatever – let it happen to me. I had a feeling that He had a plan for me and that whatever was coming would be a gift. And it happened. He gave me the gift of cancer. It's taken me a while to be able to call it that, but I see now the beauty in what's going on. He has answered a prayer I made years ago. Understanding this truth has changed my view completely on my cancer.

Before, although I didn't ask "Why me?" I was at times distraught over my diagnosis … even though I knew it was given to me for something good. It's been more than five years since my diagnosis and I have finally figured out what's going on. God has let me in on the answering of that prayer. And what am I to do with this new information? This book is a part of the answer. My great hope is that in some way my life will help not only people suffering with cancer, but more importantly suffering with life and a lack of a good relationship with God. He is the way and the truth and the life and without that inner peace knowing this, there is no way I could live my life with joy and the great love of my family.

For Steve, Rachel, Ben, Katherine and Aaron: You are the loves of my life and God has blessed me beyond measure with the gifts you are. I believe you all will go on to have beautiful, amazing lives. And I'll be praying for that.

Laura Dahl

contents

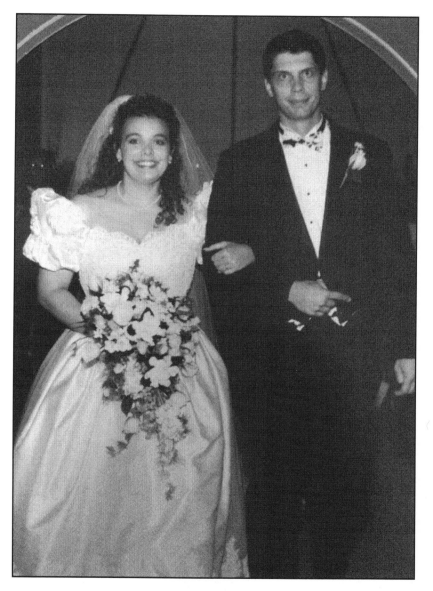

Newlyweds: Laura and Steve

and so it begins...

[14] "You are the light of the world. A city built on a hill cannot be hid. [15] No one after lighting a lamp puts it under the bushel basket, but on the lampstand, and it gives light to all in the house. [16] In the same way, let your light shine before others, so that they may see your good works and give glory to your Father in heaven.
~ Matthew 5:14-16

You may think that my cancer story should begin with my diagnosis. You wouldn't be alone if that's the case, but I just had a feeling that more had to be included to understand my story. I had to go back a little further so that people could understand and appreciate how God can work miracles, even though they might not feel like miracles at the time.

With age and hindsight, I can honestly say that I know God put my husband, Steve, and me together. My husband is a fantastic man. Loyal, honest, tall, smart, handsome... you know the type. I was lucky enough to have snagged one. We met in the first month I was at Georgia Tech. My roommate and I toured the campus hoping to meet new friends (and boys, of course). The school's man to woman ratio was 4 to 1 – good odds! About the third week into the semester, we discovered that a week-long event was taking place where we could meet lots of boys. I cannot overestimate the profound effect Rush Week had on us. Though we went to many fraternities, we ended up staying mostly with the Delta Sigs. And did we have fun! I enjoyed the parties, but the boy I was interested in was not a frat boy. I met him before school actually started at freshman orientation and, after that, no other boys had a chance ... that year, anyway. My roommate really fell for a Delta Sig guy, a couple years older than us. I thought he was nice enough, too, and oh my, did he have a nice body! That whole first year flew by and although I actually had to work to get decent grades now (a big difference from high school), I loved college.

It turned out that neither my roommate, nor the boy I was friends with returned to Tech the next year, so I started to hang out at the frat house and became better friends with the boy the other girl liked – Steve. The rest, as they say, is history! I won't say that our relationship went really smoothly (mostly because I was a brat and wasn't fond of the lack of appropriate girlfriend attention from Steve). After we graduated, we both realized a serious decision needed to be made about our intentions. For me, it was a no-brainer. I had known that Steve was the one for quite some time. He, on the other hand, needed some convincing and because we were living in two separate states, I decided to move to Louisiana to be with him and solidify the marriage thing. About a year later, on September 10, 1994, we were married.

We moved to Birmingham, Alabama for a couple of years and then to Melbourne, Florida, where my parents lived. Although you'd think living in Florida would be dreamy, it was not without issues. But we did meet some wonderful and dear friends there - Mike and Beth Paulson. They had just moved down from New York State to work at the same company where Steve worked, and we quickly became quite close. They are a truly amazing couple – wicked smart, kind, strong – and caught on quickly to the game: Canasta! We taught them how to play, being the super intelligent people they are. We played girls versus guys, thank goodness, so the odds evened up a bit. They came over almost every Saturday night for dinner and the game. Since we've moved, many people have asked me how I learned to cook so well. That's easy, Beth Paulson. To this day, with a job and three busy children, she's gourmet all the way. I, on the other hand, have had to cut back some on that and we frequently eat – freezer gourmet (pizza) or Sam's gourmet (frozen flounder… good!). We lived in Florida close to Mike and Beth for five years before making the difficult decision to move to Illinois. In another God-incident, we remain friends even though they made the move to Massachusetts a couple of years after we moved to Illinois. They are God parents to two of our children, Ben and Katherine, and stay in touch often. Mike and Beth are forever friends.

Moving to Illinois was bittersweet. We knew it was going to be a huge change from Central Florida, not the least being the weather. We ended up in Mahomet (in central Illinois) in early October and it had already started to cool off. In the first week, I found the Land's End store and bought a lavender winter coat. It was a tad puffy, (more like a down comforter) but, and this is critical, warm! I was wearing it outside later that month when the temperatures got down into the low forties. These temps only went down further, of course. My first Midwest winter was not what I had mentally prepared for when I told Steve "it'll be fine," and "We're not staying real long, right?!" The second winter, still grey and cold to the bones, had me talking to the doctors about anti-depressants. I did end up with the meds and used them for the first couple of winters. My mother called it "better living through chemistry." And they did help me a lot. I decided not to take them after 2003, though, after attending my first Cursillo and getting more into Jesus and less into me. But last winter was really tough and I thought about asking the doctor about getting some for this winter, but it's gone by so fast, I haven't needed them so far.

As I write this in February 2014, I am considering my next move, both medically and spiritually. Primary on my list is to finish this book. My goal is to be done by spring break in March. No more procrastinating! For a long time God has been pointing me toward working with hunger and I recently read a book I really want to share with friends. "7 - An Experimental Mutiny Against Excess" by Jen Hatmaker. I know it's something we can do and I am eager to start, but this book needs to be done, and it will be. Thank you Jesus for the push to finish!

in the right direction

Earth's crammed with heaven,
And every common bush afire with God,
But only he who sees takes off his shoes;
The rest sit round and pluck blackberries.
~ Elizabeth Barrett Browning

After my Cursillo weekend in November 2003, my life literally changed. During that weekend, God showed me what Love really meant; how much He loved me and, with this new relationship, what He was looking for. Clearly, I needed to spread the Good News, needed to act out my new-found love for God. Not being experienced at such a life, I started with what I did know – cooking. The local Cursillo chapter usually holds four weekends a year, two women's and two men's, and it took a lot of work - a tremendous amount of work. I was happy to work hours a day annually serving the ladies and gentlemen going through each Cursillo, and since my talents really came in the kitchen, that's where I put most of my time and energy, sometimes working for 12 hours a day during the weekend.

My Cursillo life did eventually start to slow down in 2005 with the birth of beautiful Katherine. It was still a crucial part of my life, I just had to cut back somewhat now that we had three children. And then our littlest blessing came two years later with the birth of Aaron. He was a bit of a surprise, but an amazing blessing. God knew exactly what our family was supposed to look like and the four children, Rachel, Ben, Katherine and Aaron, felt so right. We knew we needed an even amount anyway. Steve and I have always loved amusement park rides and he actually joked that having an evenly distributed family is a must for rides such as Pirates of the Caribbean and Space Mountain at Disneyworld.

Church was always a part of our lives, but after my Cursillo and then especially after Steve went through Cursillo, it became much more central. No more missing mass and holy days. I still was holding on to a simple view of what church meant, but we were faithful and thankfully God has shown me how it's really about us. He doesn't need church, I do. Now I realize I need church more than ever. And, as a bonus, I think my family needs it, too. It's the place where we can meet Jesus personally and where we can receive the Eucharist and all of our blessings directly from Him.

Our local church is Our Lady of the Lake and since we became parishioners, we have had two pastors, both of whom I love. First was Father Horton. We had been going to this parish since moving to Mahomet back in 2001, but after Cursillo, I knew we all needed to know more about our faith. When I joined my first Bible study in the winter of 2004, this fact became abundantly clear. I arrived early to the first meeting and I started talking to Fr. Horton. Just before the class began, he turned to me and said "I'm sorry, but...who are you?" Two plus years of going to this church and the pastor was just now learning my name … not exactly how you want things to start off, but since then, my learning has been such a blessing. Religious study is something a lot of people miss, thinking they got it when they were young in Sunday school. But that's just the start. Once you start reading the Bible, you realize how much more you need to learn, and how much is out there. A great place to start is a Bible study at your church, and also reading books from the local religious book store. At the end of this book, I have listed some of the books I've read that have really moved me and increased my understanding.

Looking back now, I realize how much God put in front of me to read so that my faith would continue to strengthen in order to handle the great struggle ahead.

Our second pastor came to our church a few years ago after Father Horton retired. His name is Monsignor Ramer and he has been a great leader for our church. I got along well with Father Horton and I get along well with Monsignor Ramer. I made a specific point to get to know both of these pastors by inviting them to dinner at least once a month. I also made sure I invited them to holiday dinners. Somebody told me that often these pastors spend their Christmas or Thanksgiving dinners at home alone. Since that first Cursillo and my dawn of true Christian awareness, it has included both pastors. I feel like I was blind and now I can see.

Laura Dahl

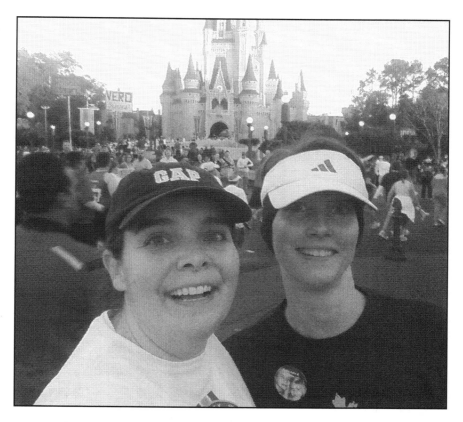

Laura and Karen - January 10, 2009 – Disney Half Marathon

the best vacation ever!

Do not regret growing old, it's a privilege denied many.
~ Anonymous

February 15, 2008

So, it's my birthday. 38 years old. I know people say this all the time, but where the hell did the time go?

I decided I needed to accomplish something before I turned 40. Yes, I know I had four beautiful children, a successful marriage, friends, etc. etc. etc. But I'd never really challenged myself on any kind of grand scale. Now, some of you might not think this qualifies as "grand," but I decided to sign up for the Disney Half Marathon scheduled for the following January. Had I ever done one? No. Had I ever run more than one mile in my entire 38 years? No. Was I in any kind of shape whatsoever that made me think I could do this... far from it! I was inspired by my husband, his sister and her husband who had run in several

Laura Dahl

full marathons and half marathons. As you may have already figured out, they were (and still are) in much better shape than me. But, no matter, I was going to do it! I signed up and paid my $140 – I was 100% committed!

Fast forward four months. My sister-in-law, who decided she was going to run the race with me, called and asked what my mile-time was. Um, well, I haven't exactly timed it yet. How many miles are you running each week? Um, well, what exactly do you mean by "running?" If you mean walking at a fairly fast pace around the block once or twice a week, then I guess about one mile. Yep, it was way past time to get serious. The date, January 10, 2009, was looming and I was really afraid I wouldn't be able to walk 13.2 miles, let alone run it. But, I got started on a 13-week walk-run program, found in The Beginning Runner's Handbook by Ian MacNeill and the Sport Medicine Council of British Columbia. This took me to the level that I could run a 10k. If you're counting, that means I only had about two and a half months left to run an additional seven miles. By the end of December, I was running for ten miles straight, no stopping. I use the word "running" loosely, because I was really just trotting at a 13-minute mile pace. But you know what they say - slow and steady wins the race. Well, I didn't intend on winning, but I did plan to finish. I felt fantastic and alive and so impressed with myself. I was really going to do it!

Just about this time I went to have a massage because, well, I deserved one. Secondarily, my back had really started to bother me, especially my lower back. So I took advantage of my parents being in town for Christmas and went over to our little local spa one day for some "me" time. The therapist showed me to the room and instructed me to undress, lay face down on the table and that she would be back in a few minutes. In happy anticipation of an hour of pure bliss, I quickly followed instructions, but when I lay down on my front side, a quick sharp pain in my left breast broke the mood. Although the massage itself was great and the pain subsided, the sharpness of it made me wonder what it could possibly be.

Apparently, I can't connect dots very well, as five months previously I had discovered something weird in my breast – not a lump, but a thickening, like a firmer section on the left side of the left breast. When at my one year post partum appointment in August of 2008, I asked the nurse practitioner about it, she cautiously dismissed it but told me to have a mammogram in January adding "it's about time for us to get a baseline, anyway." I walked out of that office without another thought about my breast, except when it started to hurt sometime in late November or early December – not all the time - just the occasional twinge which felt a lot like the beginning of a case of mastitis. This I thought was a little odd since I hadn't been breastfeeding Aaron for 6 months.

In the meantime, I continued to train and by the end of December I was up to 10 miles - an enormous accomplishment for me, the chubby girl who had never run more than a mile in her life. My back was aching, but I thought no pain no gain! I was tired a lot, but felt that the stress on my body of running that much was totally worth it. On January 9th 2009 the six of us boarded a plane for one of the best vacations we have ever had at Disney World, blissfully unaware that life as we knew it would radically change forever just a couple of weeks later.

Laura Dahl

on my knees

There are two ways to live your life:
one is as though nothing is a miracle,
the other is as though everything is a miracle.
~ Albert Einstein

Ever had a moment when time seems to stand still? You know, like when your boyfriend asks you to marry him, or when your favorite team wins the championship game at the last second, or when you hold your newborn child and look into her eyes for the first time. These moments implant themselves indelibly in our brains, never ever to leave. All these beautiful moments I have experienced myself and they live in my memory almost as vividly as when they originally happened. Thank God for these cherished events and the subsequent memories they create! Unfortunately, we all know that life isn't filled only with cheery and gay, sunshine on your shoulders kind of moments. Time stands still for the dark moments too.

So, we got back from our incredible vacation, and I was on

Laura Dahl

top of the world and feeling like I could accomplish anything, almost… invincible. As I looked at my calendar, I realized that I had my mammogram scheduled for early the following week. Good, I thought, I'll get that done and over with and then I can plan my next race. I wasn't scared walking into the newly erected building and I don't remember being fazed at all by the name of the building – Carle Cancer Center. I was not even worried about the squishing that my breasts were about to undergo (although lots of women like to describe how awful it is, it's really not that bad – really). I walked out after my appointment ready to move on. A few days later though, while I was in the pick up line at my daughter's preschool, the nurse practitioner called to say there were "calcifications" – whatever they were – that showed up on the mammogram. She assured me that there was no lump, and there wasn't anything to be overly concerned about, but I would need to have a biopsy to be sure. Two things went through my mind, the first more pronounced than the second – crap, when am I going to have time to get that done? … and then, biopsy? That doesn't sound good. I was scheduled for the procedure for Monday afternoon, only a few days later. Steve came with me for moral support and afterward, still smarting (yeah, a needle biopsy stings quite a bit) we went to get ice cream and soothed our anxiety with sweet, creamy goodness.

The Worst Day

I can remember, with almost perfect clarity, the day I learned I had cancer. You know when you're waiting for test results and you answer the phone and your doctor is on the other end, it's probably not going to be good news. I was in my kitchen, my youngest child napping peacefully upstairs, when I got my call. As soon as I heard her voice, I was filled with dread. She attempted to make the usual small talk "Hi, how are you?" but she quickly moved on to the purpose of her call.

"I'm so sorry to have to tell you this, but your biopsy came back positive for Ductal Carcinoma In Situ." That sounds pretty bad, right? I mean I had no idea what 'In Situ' meant, but I sure as heck knew what carcinoma meant. To her credit, the doctor was quite caring and gentle on the phone, asking me several times if I was okay (clearly not) and if I had anyone at home (well, yes, my 19 month old, who was blessedly still snoozing during this overwhelming phone call). She said she was sorry to have given me such news over the phone, but correctly assumed I would have worried much more about why she was calling me in had she made me schedule an appointment. As you might imagine, at this point I was barely able to hold myself up. She finally asked if she could call someone for me and, in a very small voice that was barely audible, I whispered "No, no, that's okay," and hung up. And fell to my knees, bawling out loud, completely overcome by the shock of this word which, prior to this call, I hadn't given very much thought to at all, but which now became a part of who I am. Cancer.

Such an ugly sounding word, don't you think? I guess that's because it's so ubiquitous and carries so much meaning for such a simple word. Cancer. Just saying it brings to mind all sorts of other scary words: pain, suffering, hospital, chemotherapy, radiation, death. But those are just words people use to describe an awful disease that happens to other people. When it's you, what happens on the inside is very hard to describe, there are no words – only this feeling of melting. This is clearly not to be confused with the gooey, warm feeling one gets when falling in

Laura Dahl

love. For example, "my heart melted when he gave me a ring." Oh no, this melting is when, upon hearing the news, your body feels like there is no longer anything supporting it; like everything is collapsing in on itself. Thank God for small miracles – my son continued to sleep during my emotional melt down and didn't have to see his mother, a puddle of goo, sobbing on the kitchen floor. As I began to come back to myself, but still teary and breathing like a toddler who'd just come out of a temper tantrum, I knew I had to make some phone calls.

The first call was to my husband, who was, of course, out of town for the day. When he answered, I just blurted out "It's cancer! The biopsy results came back and it's cancer." After releasing a hard breath, he told me that everything would be alright and that he would come home as fast as he could and that he loved me. Yes, he is a great guy and I am extraordinarily thankful to have married him. After talking to him, I had to calm down enough to make the next call, Mom. I had called her the week before to tell her about the mammogram results and ask her what "calcifications" were and what the biopsy would entail. She had just gone through this process a few years earlier and her results were good. When I called that day, I think she already knew that the news would be grim because there was no shock in her response, just sadness. She was a nurse back in her working days and knew that patients frequently don't recall what the doctors tell them. She asked me again what my doctor had told me. "It was Ductal Carcinoma In Situ, Mom – that's what she said." I'm not sure if she knew what the 'In Situ' part meant either, but that didn't matter, it was the carcinoma part that stunned us both to the core.

How was it possible that I should have cancer? My stats were pretty good, although admittedly I could have lost 30 pounds or so. I'm a non-smoker, non-drinker (occasional glasses of wine notwithstanding), no recent birth control pill use. I breast fed all four of my children. I had just run a half marathon. I was 38 years old, for Pete's sake! Young women don't get breast cancer, right? I wasn't supposed to get cancer!

In hind sight, of course, I should have been much more vigilant. I already mentioned my mother's close call, but my family tree is filled with relatives stricken with cancer. Apparently, my grandmother (Dad's side) had breast cancer back in the late seventies, had a mastectomy and never had a recurrence. My aunt (Mom's side) had fairly recently been diagnosed with stage 1 breast cancer but passed away in January of 2012. My other aunt died from lung cancer, as well as her father, and my grandma died from colon cancer. But they were all smokers, or heavily exposed to smoke in my Grandma's case – decades of inhaling carcinogenic garbage. So I can see that connection. Smoking = Cancer, right? Cancer was just not on the radar screen as something that I had to be concerned about and all this family history just got filed away.

After I got that call on February 5, 2009, things began to happen very quickly, no time to let the news settle or to try come to terms with the facts. I got another call from the doctor's office later that afternoon that we had appointments the next day with an oncologist, a radiation oncologist, and a surgeon. My husband and I were sent to the Mills Breast Cancer Center at our local hospital for our appointments. I say our, because from the moment I told him the news, my husband had breast cancer too. And, except for work, we were inseparable.

The breast cancer nurse came in to our exam room and began to very quickly go over a large folder with lots of papers and glossy brochures – kind of like we were being welcomed into some sort of club – "welcome to the world of cancer" – none of which I remember and none of which I kept. She was soon booted out when the oncologist blew in (a wisp of a man who somehow had a commanding presence anyway). He gave us the details of the biopsy report: Ductal Carcinoma In Situ Her 2 Nue +++/ ER+1%/PR-. Translation: the cancer had not left the Ductal walls (great news) but was highly aggressive (bad news). The doctor went on to describe the process to come: surgery to remove the affected breast tissue, then radiation to make sure any cells which might have escaped the knife were taken care of. Then he happily pronounced that this was considered stage 0 Cancer and had a 90% cure rate. Now, that sounds really, really good looking back, but at the time, I was horrified about that remaining 10%.

The surgeon was very kind and went over my options, I could have a mastectomy, but that really wasn't called for in my situation so he recommended a lumpectomy. He carefully explained that he would remove the area where the mammogram had shown calcifications plus a little extra to ensure clean margins. There would be a noticeable "divet" in my breast, he told us, but at this point I was ready for him to just cut the whole damn thing off.

Our third and final doctor consult of the day was with the radiation oncologist. Standard treatment was six weeks of radiation treatments, one per day not including the weekends. He explained in great detail what he was going to do. He even drew a diagram to show us how tricky treating the left breast is due to the location of the heart, because you know that could present a problem irradiating my heart. Yes, danger is clear now doctor, thank you. But wait, there's more … he paused after explaining all this and then looked at my husband and me with a seriousness that made my blood run cold. He had reviewed the mammogram report and images and was concerned about a few things. Although the mammogram just showed calcifications, the radiologist who performed the biopsy and wrote the report was concerned about the large, dense blotch showing on the far left side and recommended a breast MRI to clarify. The radiation oncologist discussed this with us and recommended the same. I was scheduled for an MRI the next week.

An MRI creates highly detailed images using powerful magnets and uses no radiation. It sees much more than a traditional x-ray (which is essentially what a mammogram is) and boy, did it find all kinds of nasty stuff in my case. I went to my doctor appointment the following week by myself – I had done a pretty good job of reassuring myself that I was going to be cured; that in six weeks all this cancer crap would be over. I didn't need anyone to come with me. I was going to be fine. That was the last appointment I went to alone.

My doctor, the cheery medical oncologist we had met a couple of weeks earlier, was not smiling. He looked at me with somber eyes. He told me that the MRI results showed a very small 4mm tumor with DCIS (Ductal Carcinoma In Situ) in more than half my breast, and many lymph nodes which were extraordinarily large. Without really explaining anything, just stating he was "very concerned" and that he wanted to wait to make the next move until after my genetic testing came back, he left the room. All confidence lost, scared and confused, I fled the office and drove home. And, of course, my husband was out of town again. Thank God my best friend, Christy Madura, was at my house when I got back – she had been babysitting my little guy. I just fell into her arms and cried. I had never been so scared in my entire life and I will be forever grateful she was there to listen and to help me calm down. I knew this new development was bad – really bad.

The radiation oncologist wanted to see me about this, too. Thankfully, my husband was with me for this appointment. It's amazing how much I realized during these early days how very desperately I needed him. He is rock solid, and his loyalty and integrity are amazing. Most importantly, he loves me. After almost 15 years of marriage, I was still his main squeeze. He took those vows seriously "in sickness and in health." The doctor told us the results and explained that this meant that clearly a lumpectomy and radiation were out. More ominously, he was very concerned about those lymph nodes. I didn't know it at the time, but what he was concerned about was that the cancer had already spread outside my breast. My only choice at this point was whether to have a single or double mastectomy and then, whether or not I wanted to have reconstructive surgery. Both doctors agreed that we should wait to schedule any surgery until the results of genetic testing came back. I, however, had already decided on a double mastectomy. I didn't want to take any chances. As reality started to sink in, I figured that since they had served their purpose in breast-feeding my children, they were goners. I've never been particularly fond of my breasts anyway – too big and, now too droopy. After meeting with a plastic surgeon about reconstruction surgery, I was actually kinda excited about getting a new set! Trying to look on the bright side, nice new perky boobs seemed like pretty good compensation for having cancer!

At some point during these doctor appointments, I mentioned to the nurse that my back, which had been bothering me for the last couple of months had really started to hurt. She chalked it up to stress and I chalked it up to the running, though I had not done any running since returning from vacation just four weeks prior. She talked to my oncologist and he immediately scheduled a bone scan. They explained that I would be injected with a sugary radioactive tracer and then scanned to see if any of the tracer was "taken up" in any bones. At this point, my hope started to sag and after the scan, I really started to have a bad feeling about my situation and my suspicions grew. I came to the realization, though not yet a full understanding, that if this scan report came back showing any activity, I was in real danger. Mortal danger.

The Second Worst Day
(Really, THE VERY WORST DAY)

On February 25, 2009, Steve and I went to the Cancer Center for an appointment with the surgeon (whom we knew because he had performed Steve's appendectomy several years before). We waited in the small lobby just outside the exam rooms. My dread was palpable and my husband could tell that something was wrong. As we walked into the exam area, I whispered to him, "I've got a really bad feeling about this. I think my bone scan is going to show something," and we turned to walk into our little room. As the surgeon was about to come in, my oncologist squeezed in ahead of the guy, told him he needed to see us for a minute and shut the door. At that moment, I knew there would be no mastectomy, there would be no perky new set of breasts. I remember looking at my husband and trying to absorb some of his strength and when he looked back at me, there was fear in his eyes that I had never seen before. The doctor proceeded to go over the results from the bone scan and, boy, was it bad. There were likely metastases to the pelvis, sternum, right scapula, lumbar spine, thoracic spine, skull and possibly the right femur. The worst fear a cancer patient faces when they are diagnosed at stage 1, 2, or 3 is that someday the cancer may progress into stage 4 - Terminal. That's where I was now. Only three short weeks ago, I was a curable stage 0, but now dying rapidly at stage 4.

I valiantly tried to hold in the sobs, but then Steve asked what this meant as far as my prognosis went. The doctor quietly replied, "Well it's not for sure, but maybe one to two years." This was followed by my immediate meltdown. I was sobbing without abandon; barely able to sit on the exam table; with Steve wrapping his arms around me. Was he crying? Maybe, but I was crying enough for the two of us anyway. I finally stopped sobbing long enough, but still crying hard, to tell him over and over "I'm sorry. I'm so sorry." And then, "The kids, oh my God, the kids! Katherine and Aaron won't even remember me!" And then, after much more crying and "I'm sorry's," the doctor sent the social worker/therapist in to talk to us and my sobs began to subside. She asked some questions, none of which I could answer and none of which I even remember. My mind kept repeating the names of my husband and children. What were we going to do? I was going to die from this. My children would grow up without their mother and my husband would be a young widower. He would have to somehow continue working and single-handedly raise our four children, then aged 11, 8, 3, and 19 months. These thoughts consumed me and were intensely painful. My heart ached more than I ever thought it could and I was filled with an all-consuming sorrow. This was different from the melting experience of the day I found out I had cancer. That was a day of crying for me;

that was me being sorry for myself. This pain was way beyond that. It was for the people that I loved so dearly in this world. I was feeling sorry for them.

My two youngest were at home when we got back from the doctor and I snatched them both up and hugged them as never before, realizing how very precious they and their older brother and sister were to me. I quietly cried while Steve showed our kind neighbor who was watching them to the door. I could think of nothing but my family and when the two older children came home I embraced them too, feeling such an intense amount of love that I almost started bawling again. I think we only made two phone calls that day – I called my best friend, Christy, and Steve called his sister, Karen, who happens to be a doctor. I just knew that mentally, physically, and emotionally, we could not make any other calls that day. That day, Ash Wednesday, February 25, 2009, was the single worst day in my life.

The next day I called my sister at home because at that time my Dad was living with her while working. He and my Mom actually lived a couple hours north from my sister, and he normally went home for the weekends, but during the week my mother was alone. My father had not left for work yet that morning (another bit of Divine Providence because he usually left early). I told my sister that she should sit down, but, being the loving, rather demanding little sister that she was, she insisted I tell her right away. I told her that the cancer had spread to my bones – now stage 4 - and that I needed her and Dad to drive up to Jacksonville to be with Mom before I called. There was no way I was giving her this kind of news while she was alone. She put Dad on the phone and after I told him, I could tell he was upset, not crying, but very quiet. He then agreed to leave immediately to be with Mom.

When I called her, she took the news hard, but in a graceful way that gave me some strength. When I told her I was sorry to bring this on her, she immediately ordered me not to apologize that this was not something I did and had nothing to be sorry for. Still, and even to this day, I remain sorry for causing my loved ones so much pain.

A week or two earlier, at the suggestion of my best friend who was getting a steady stream of phone calls from friends and fellow parishioners asking about me, I started posting information on Caring Bridge, a free online journaling site. The site allowed me to post what was going on and my best friend to get some peace. On February 26, 2009, I wrote this:

"Everybody take a deep breath with me and hang on – this road just got a lot bumpier. Had the worst day of my life yesterday when we learned that it appears the cancer has spread to my bones. The bone scan shows "hot spots" in the skull, spine, sternum, pelvis, right scapula and possibly the right femur. This would mean that I am stage IV. I am having a better day today, but yesterday was really hard. I think God was preparing me for those results because I really had a strong feeling the scan would come back positive. In fact, just before we went back to see the doctor I told Steve that I felt that the news wasn't going to be good.

The doctor ordered a brain MRI and CT scan of my torso to see if the cancer has spread to any soft tissue. Got those out of the way this morning and they weren't too bad - just had to drink the nastiest liquid for the CT scan, blech!

Surgery has been put on the back burner for now as this new problem is a greater threat. I find out my results from these 2 scans tomorrow when we meet with the oncologist again. We'll also decide on the next step - probably a biopsy so we can determine the best treatment plan.

Please continue to pray for a miracle for me and strength for Steve. He has been wonderful - my rock - and in many ways his role in all this will be much more difficult than my own. Also pray for my family - this is so hard on them too. I just HATE that I am causing them so much pain. And of course, my children - pray that they stay strong through this whole process and still can enjoy just being kids. Every time I think about how this will affect them I start to cry, so pray that I can be strong for them too.

There is still hope, and I am trying very hard to remain positive. I am definitely feeling God's presence and I know He will be right here with me no matter what."

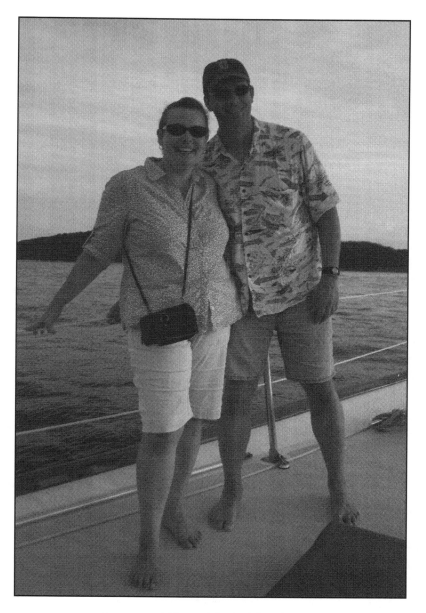

Laura and Steve, Virgin Islands, 2009

what now?

It's not the load that brings you down;
it's how you carry it
~ Lena Horne

Looking back, it seems to me that the whole month of February flew by in the blink of an eye. Things happened so fast, so many doctor appointments, so many tests, so many bad reports. But in all that time, by the beginning of March there were still unanswered questions, still more tests to be done, and still no treatment. I was very frustrated that the pace had seemingly slowed to snail speed. All the while, the pain was getting worse and my fears consistently gnawed at my nerves. My doctor ordered several scans – a brain MRI and a CTscan and a bone biopsy to confirm the diagnosis of metastatic disease, and to confirm the type of breast cancer I had. I came to learn later that there are at least 15 different kinds of breast cancer. The biggest confirmation he needed was regarding the Her2+++ status. Because there are so many kinds of cancer, each one has its own starting approach, but if mine proved to be Her2 positive, the direction to go was clear. There was a clinical trial that included a recently FDA approved drug which specifically targets Her2+ breast cancer. Here's a great explanation about Her2 positive breast cancer and the new drug, from the Mayo Clinic website:

HER2-positive breast cancer is a breast cancer that tests positive for a protein called human epidermal growth factor receptor 2 (HER2), which promotes the growth of cancer cells. In about 1 of every 5 breast cancers, the cancer cells make an excess of HER2 due to a gene mutation. This gene mutation and the elevated levels of HER2 that it causes can occur in many types of cancer — not only breast cancer. This is a gene mutation that occurs only in the cancer cells and is not a type of mutation that you can inherit from a parent.

HER2-positive breast cancers tend to be more aggressive than other types of breast cancer. They're also less responsive to hormone treatment. However, treatments that specifically target HER2 are very effective. They include:

• **Trastuzumab (Herceptin)**. *Trastuzumab, which specifically targets HER2, kills these cancer cells and decreases the risk of recurrence. Trastuzumab is often used with chemotherapy. But it may also be used alone or in combination with hormone-blocking medications, such as an aromatase inhibitor or tamoxifen. Trastuzumab is usually well tolerated, but it does have some potential side effects, such as congestive heart failure and allergic reaction.*
http://www.mayoclinic.com/health/breast-cancer/AN00495

The brain MRI came back great. The report read "unremarkable brain" which I was completely happy with and with which Steve had lots of fun. The CT scan came back showing a small 1cm spot on my liver, but the doctor dismissed it saying it was too small to say what it might be. On March 11th, I received the bone biopsy that showed that I was indeed Her2 positive. It was official – I had stage IV breast cancer. I spoke with the doctor the following week to make the treatment plan. In everything I'd read, and on the advice of my mother and sister-in-law (the doctor) I wanted to get a second opinion and because my sister-in-law, Karen, had gone to medical school at Washington University in St. Louis and it was only three hours from home, I made an appointment to see a Dr. Bose who specialized in Her2 positive breast cancers. We saw him on Friday, March 20th and he was very kind, spent a lot of time with us and recommended the same thing as had Dr. Rowland. After we left his office, we went back to the hotel to get ready for dinner. At 5:30 p.m. I heard my phone ring. It was Dr. Bose and he had just received the report on the blood sample I had given hours earlier. They showed alarmingly high liver numbers. He told us that I should have another CT scan ASAP and not to wait long to start treatment. I had planned on getting a third opinion in Chicago but that seemed unnecessary because both oncologists I had already seen agreed on the same treatment plan. We all went up to Chicago, anyway, just to have some sorely needed fun. Unfortunately, it didn't last long for me.

On Monday morning, I called the nurse back at my home hospital to get the results from the PET scan I'd gotten done the Friday morning before leaving for St. Louis. The results were really ugly and scary, and I started to fear for my life. Spots were lighting up in my liver, ovaries, adrenal glands, and lungs in addition to my left breast and a dozen or so lymph nodes – things had gotten seriously ugly in a very short period of time, really a few weeks. I made arrangements with her to have a medi-port surgically installed the next day (Tuesday 3/24), which sounds a little weird but it's been a huge blessing. The doctor put the medi-port just under the skin placed just below my right collarbone with a tube running from the port to a large vein near my heart. I got to test drive the new port the following day to start treatment, not at my home hospital, but down in St. Louis. My local doctor was on vacation that week and therefore couldn't write any orders, but I told the nurse I could not wait one more week to begin, that I needed treatment four weeks ago. No, I could, would not wait. Dr. Bose graciously allowed me to start treatment at Wash U/Barnes Cancer Center and, although it took a long time and I had some negative reactions, I got the first dose of the drugs that would work wonders. This was seven long weeks after that first call from my OB/GYN. I still can't believe how long it took to get the first treatment.

the power of prayer

Those who are wise will shine like the brightness
of the heavens, and those who lead many to
righteousness, like the stars for ever and ever.
~ Daniel 12:3 (NIV)

I thought I had a pretty good handle on my faith before cancer became a part of my life. I went to Mass regularly, including most Holy Days and went to confession less often than I should have, but still made it at least once a year. I was a good, faithful Catholic girl, especially after the Cursillo in 2003, when I got the wake-up call from God that my relationship with Him was shallow and I needed to draw close to Him and stay there. He knew what was coming down the road and how spiritually ill-prepared I was. That Cursillo weekend, He made Himself so present to me that I heard His call loud and clear. Wake up from your slumber, girl! I gave my life for you! I love you unconditionally!

One of the most important things I learned in 2003 was how

to have an active prayer life. There is no way to develop a relationship with Him other than by communicating. I began to pray and study and actively try to make a difference in this world.

Prayer, I think, is hard for a lot of people. It was hard for me before I attended Cursillo, and I still had to consistently work at it. An active prayer life doesn't happen overnight. I prayed every evening and throughout the day as I read and heard about different prayer requests. And I studied, reading a lot of spiritual books, starting off with Mere Christianity by C.S. Lewis and many books about Mother Teresa. But I still wasn't where I needed to be. I was still having trouble turning away from myself, turning toward others and putting their concerns ahead of mine. I was still letting the busyness of life take me away from my relationship building with the most important Person in my life. But there's nothing like a swift kick in the pants to get you serious about your faith… a kick like getting diagnosed with a life-threatening illness!

I keep going back to that Cursillo weekend in 2003 because I know it was God's plan to prepare me for what was coming. During that retreat weekend I heard much talk about faith and Christianity, but one talk in particular struck a major chord for some reason. It was given by a Non-Denominational minister who also happened to be a recovering alcoholic. Two things were indelibly etched into my heart and soul from his story: 1) To get serious about prayer, you best do it on your knees, and 2) When someone asks you to do something spiritual, just say yes! These are the two doctrines he lived by on his successful road to recovery, sobriety and living a life devoted to Christ. I live by them now, too, though I have to admit it hasn't always been easy. I haven't always said yes, but I try and my life is so much richer, so much better, my faith is so much stronger, my love is so much bigger for having prayed on my knees and said Yes!

Yes, God was preparing me for this trial. Without my strong faith I would not have been able to get back up off my kitchen floor that awful February morning or to recover from finding out I was stage IV later that month; that someday, sooner rather than later, this disease would probably steal my life. My relationship with Jesus has been such a huge part of my life since then, I am amazed. I could not have imagined being here today, more than five years later, writing a memoir about my experiences. I have leaned on Him every day. I thank Him every day... for my life and for the untold blessings I have. "The LORD is compassionate and gracious, Slow to anger and abounding in loving kindness." Psalm 103:8

"Joy Manifesto" 4/17/2009 from personal diary, my first entry – nobody else has read until now:

The last couple of months have been pretty bad. That's probably an understatement – the worst in my life would be more accurate. I have been diagnosed with breast cancer which has metastasized to my bones, liver, lungs, and various other spots in my abdomen. Yeah, probably an understatement. Up until February 5, 2009, my life was pretty darn picture perfect. Wonderful husband of 14 ½ years, 4 beautiful children, nice house, great job (stay at home mom), fantastic church community and many friends (etc, etc, etc). For some years now, I've been waiting for the other shoe to drop. "It can't possibly be this good and last" I would say to myself. I would pray that should something bad happen, "please God, let it be me and not my children." Well, be careful what you pray for right? In all seriousness though, one of the things I have been most thankful for during this whole process is that it is me and not one of my children, I'm certain I couldn't handle that. One of my favorite quotes is from Mother Teresa "I know God won't give me anything I can't handle, I just wish He didn't trust me so much." He obviously knew I could somehow handle cancer happening to me, but also knows I couldn't function if something had happened to one of my kids.

As this whole mess has unfolded, however, the one dominating thought I've had has been how wonderful my life really is. I have known such joy and been filled with so much love and I know nothing can change that fact. Having a life-threatening illness has only magnified my awareness of that fact. I look at the world very differently now. Each morning I wake up to my dear husband and hear birds chirping, I thank God for another day in my own little paradise. I see beauty in the simplest of God's creations – daffodils so sunshiny yellow that you can't help but feel happy looking at them; clear blue sunny days; the sound of birds chirping; the smell of freshly cut grass. I now treasure each and every day and I'm determined to find joy in them – whether I've got just a handful of days left or thousands. Actually, finding joy has been remarkably easy. The purpose of this journal is to make sure I remember them and to let the people I love know how much joy I felt each day. Thank you God for the incredible amount of joy you've given me in this life."

end of chemo

Somewhere over the rainbow,
Skies are blue,
And the dreams that you dare to dream
Really do come true.
~ Lyman Frank Baum

Those early days of cancer were filled with every kind of emotion a human being can have: terror, impatience, sorrow, pain, loneliness, joy, peace, trust and security. While the negative emotions definitely ruled, there were some really great days when cancer lost the battle for my soul. God was the One who saved me from my own wretchedness. In His Love is power and I felt it then and now. He worked through friends, sending me lots of Bible verses. Some of my favorites were Joshua 1:9, Sirach 2:1-11 – all directing me to put my trust in the Lord. For me, there was no other way to live.

While chemotherapy was difficult, it wasn't the horror that I had heard and read about, and the cancer responded very well to the cocktail I was receiving. By late May 2009, my CT scan showed no evidence of disease in the ovaries, adrenal glands or lungs and the largest liver lesion had been reduced by half. The good reports kept coming in, finally, and that was really heartening, especially after receiving such bad news for weeks on end! By the end of my treatment on September 3rd, all signs pointed to a great outcome from the treatment I received. And I was so excited to be done. I wrote on Caring Bridge:

Yay!!!!! I'm DONE - final chemo yesterday!...

It's so amazing to look back over the last 6 months - it was long at times but ironically, it flew by too. I am so incredibly grateful for all the love and support you all have given to me and my family. It would have been an impossible journey without your help and your prayers lifted us up in such a beautiful way. "Thank you" seems so inadequate, but I guess those are the only words we've got - know that you all are in our daily prayers and that we love you! I also want to mention how wonderful my care has been at Carle - the nurses over there are THE BEST!

This is not the end of my treatments, but we are hoping that I won't need chemotherapy again. I'll keep updating this blog as it continues. Of course, I have those scans coming up next Friday and an appointment with Dr. Rowland on the 14th so I'll update after them. Praying hard for good results, but throughout this ordeal I have learned to trust God more and myself less :-) I have repeated daily Sirach 2:6 "Trust God and He will help you. Make straight your ways and Hope in Him" and I have tried to live it. Can't say that I haven't had times of despair and anxiety, but that verse has helped me get through those rough spots.

God bless you all and I hope you have a great holiday weekend!

September 3, 2009

I was pretty happy and looking forward to some form of normalcy returning to our lives. No more weekly visits to Carle, no more family visits (though, God bless them for coming to help!) It was great to think of our family getting back into our little routine ... except for one tiny, little thing. Well, two actually. Back in July, I had a second brain MRI and at the time, I didn't know that for about a third of Her2 positive patients there was a very high threat of the cancer spreading to the brain. But, they had only seen a small spot. When the nurse called with those results, she only said that there was nothing "significant" which showed up on the report. Nothing significant? What the heck does that mean? The doctor blew the report off though, saying that the radiologist who read the MRI wasn't sure and that "it could be anything." I tried to put it behind me, I really did, but of course that's hard when you know now that among people diagnosed with cancer, brain metastases are the tip of the iceberg of fear, the worst of the worst case scenarios. I sent the scan images down to St. Louis to be reviewed by the radiologist there and they dismissed that little 2mm pinpoint as nothing to be concerned about; that it could have even just been a blood vessel.

Sigh. It wasn't just a blood vessel. The MRI that I had just a week after finishing my chemo treatments, showed that the little 2mm spot was the same but another spot had popped up. I sent this scan down to St. Louis as well, hoping, praying, begging God that it wasn't what everyone suspected it was. Caring Bridge:

October 6, 2009:
The last few weeks have been really great - I am feeling so much better. I didn't realize how bad I had started to feel after all those chemo treatments. My energy level has come back and it

feels really good to be somewhat back to normal.

I talked to Dr. Bose this morning about my recent brain MRI. The radiologists at Barnes agree with the one here at Carle – those two spots are suspicious for metastases. Not really what I wanted to hear, but it's not a surprise either. He suggested I meet with a neurosurgeon to discuss my options. I will be seeing Dr. Rowland tomorrow and will see what he says. I think I'd like to go down there and at least find out what those options are and when we'll have to worry about doing something. Right now, the lesions are very small and they haven't really changed since July. I think we will be scheduling another MRI for about 4 weeks from now, so that will show how fast they are growing.

I'll post again after tomorrow's appointment. Repeating over and over again: "Be strong and take heart all you who hope in the Lord." Ps 31:25

No, not at all what I wanted to hear. But that was nothing compared with what was coming. My local doctor was still not overly concerned, though, as the spots were very small and seemed not to be growing quickly at all. He ordered another MRI for three weeks out.

the third worst day

Grant me, O Lord my God, a mind to know you,
a heart to seek you, wisdom to find you,
conduct pleasing to you, faithful perseverance in waiting for you,
and a hope of finally embracing you. Amen.
~ Prayer of St. Thomas Aquinas

I just wanted to get away – from doctors, nurses, needles, scans, cancer, I just wanted to get away from cancer. One of the, what shall I call it, benefits – no, bonuses – no, good things – (you have to look on the bright side of this whole thing and find any scrap of good that comes out of it) – one of the perks of cancer is that you get serious about a lot of things. The first is your faith, the second is your family, and the third is your dreams. I'll come back to the first two, but for now let me just talk about the third. My bucket list had a lot of places I wanted to see, and near the top was the Caribbean. Steve and I had honeymooned in Mexico on the Riviera Maya and I loved it so much. The hotel was right on the sea and our room had a gorgeous view – we had a perfect start to our marriage! I wanted to escape back to that time. I wanted to go back to those carefree days and so we decided to make a fairly quick five day trip to the US Virgin Islands. I had found a really good deal on a resort on St. Thomas and my brother-in-law (world traveler for his job) offered to use some of his frequent flyer miles to get us airfare. I think both of us were able to leave all that cancer stuff behind us in Illinois, with maybe the exception of my very close marine-style hair. It was unbelievably beautiful there. We snorkeled in the magnificent waters off St. John's Trunk Bay and in Turtle Cove (a small island cove off of St. Thomas), and we took a sunset sailboat trip, and we crashed a wedding that took place on the beach at our hotel. Steve even tolerated some shopping in Charlotte Amalie. We ate and laughed and had so much fun. It was romantic and unforgettable, and just what we needed.

Then it was back to real life, which hit us with grey skies and 40 degree weather back in Illinois. It could not have been a bigger contrast to the amazing weather in the Virgin Islands. Neither could the carefree beauty we experienced compare to the cold, hard reality of metastatic cancer. I had the next MRI on October 28, 2009. The results came 2 days later.

Caring Bridge:
October 31, 2009
We had another really tough day yesterday. Dr. Rowland went over the brain MRI and, unfortunately, it wasn't good news. The two spots from before have doubled in size (but are still pretty small - 5mm) and there are about 8 new small lesions. I have officially been diagnosed with brain mets :(. My liver function numbers all came back normal (yay!) but, since I have been having some abdominal pain, I'm going to have a CT scan next Tuesday.

After Dr. R, we met with the radiation oncologist, Dr. Spaiente, and went over the treatment plan. Starting Monday, I will be receiving whole brain radiation every day for 13 days. Because the lesions are so small, he is optimistic that this treatment will eradicate them. The side effects aren't great - brain swelling is the worst of them, so he already started me on steroids; but also hair loss, fatigue, nausea, blah, blah, blah.... Everyone's different though, so we'll just have to see.

It was very hard yesterday to stay hopeful, because this hurdle is a real doozy. I feel like my prognosis just went from bad to worse. It's interesting how in the beginning, when I was first diagnosed with DCIS (stage 0) cancer, the doctors we're very happy to tell me I had an excellent chance of being cured. Now, we don't talk about my prognosis at all. Those statistics are based on old data anyway - and I am an individual and everyone's case is different. I keep telling myself these things, trying to make sense of the incomprehensible.

Today is better, though - at least the sun is shining :). And I feel pretty darn well! And it's Halloween! The kids are very excited - Rachel is a prom queen, Ben is a skeleton, Katherine is a genie, and Aaron is a dragon. I'll try to post a picture later. We've got our pumpkins carved and candy ready - should be lots of fun!

Please especially pray for Steve, my children and my parents - to say the least, they are dealing with extremely difficult emotions right now. The kids are handling it very well actually, but we've got tough times ahead. Steve seems to be doing alright (but it's hard to tell with him) and is my ever-optimistic partner. Thank God for him!

LIFE IS GOOD - cancer will never change that fact! This is from last Thursday's Proverbs 31 Ministries and it really struck me as both beautiful and important (so many of them have been great for me lately!) The author paraphrases Luke 1:78-79:

"Because of the tender mercy of my God by which the rising sun will come to me from heaven - to shine on my darkness and in what

feels like the shadow of death to me – I will find peace."
    Luke 1:78

Notice that the post was the day after my doctor appointment. That's because I was overcome with grief again. It was yet another worst day, complete with shock, sobbing, and a boatload of anxiety – but also prayer – a lot of prayer. It was time to get even more serious about prayer and I began to pray daily on my knees for help, for my very survival. From my personal journal the night of the 30th:

"Today is a hard day. Found out this morning that there are about 10 small lesions in my brain now – there is no mistaking what's going on. I have brain mets. I am having a lot of trouble handling this news because I feel like my little Hope bubble has now burst. I am wondering how much time I have left – and feeling it will be counted in months rather than years. I hope I am wrong of course. I need a Hail Mary pass, literally. I want so much to be hopeful, especially for Steve and the kids. I recite daily Psalm 31: "Be strong and take heart all you who hope in the Lord." And have tried (and continue to try) to put my trust in God. Somehow, I know He has a plan in all this mess – I just wish I knew what it was.

Even now, in the depths of my despair, I know my life is good. My husband and children are so wonderful – I love you all so very much. Right now it feels like my heart will implode for missing you all and the lives and important events I will miss. And the pain I know I will cause if I die sooner rather than later will be so tough. It hurts so much to think about – it's so very unfair. I am praying hard that this will serve some purpose in their lives – that somehow they will be stronger, their faith will be stronger because of my illness and death. Oh God, please let them be okay – bring them Your peace and wrap

Your loving arms around them always. Amen."

I then went on to write my husband and each child a letter. Because on that day, all I felt was despair, all hope was gone for me. It was horrible.

My children would often see me praying on my knees and asked if that was necessary to talk to God. I told them no, that they could talk to God anywhere and at anytime. But for me, in the evenings before bed, I wanted to give God my complete attention and I found that praying on my knees helped me do that. So that night, I got on my knees and I cried out to God to help me and to help my family. I know that He heard me and was crying right along with me, that He knew how desperate I was to feel His Presence and Love.

"Therefore, since we have been justified by faith, we have peace* with God through our Lord Jesus Christ,a 2through whom we have gained access [by faith] to this grace in which we stand, and we boast in hope of the glory of God.b 3Not only that, but we even boast of our afflictions, knowing that affliction produces endurance, and endurance, proven character, and proven character, hope,c 5and hope does not disappoint, because the love of God has been poured out into our hearts through the holy Spirit that has been given to us." Romans 5:1-5

There's a great theological argument for why God allows suffering and evil (great explanation can be found at http://vimeo.com/9135547). Pastor Tim Keller explains the basic premise: that, because of His Love for us, He created us with the gift of free will – the ability to choose to do the right things, to choose to love and believe in Him or not. He masterfully gave this gift to us because you can't truly love somebody if you're forced to do so. Since the dawn of humanity, we've had this gift of free will, and boy, have we made a mess of it. I'm sure God always hopes that we choose His way, but of course, we don't. So He sent His only Son down to become one of us humans, and to experience all the things we do – happiness, disappointment, joy, fear, friendship, sorrow, pain, suffering, and death. So we can relate our life experiences with His. That last part is so important to me now; that somehow I can lift up my own suffering to join in the suffering of Christ has been an immeasurable help in dealing with the darkness of cancer.

I started to study this because I think this is a big stumbling block for a lot of people when it comes to faith and cancer, and one of the leading arguments for atheism. At the time, my brother, Joey, called himself an agnostic, but he was really leaning towards atheism – a complete lack of belief. He didn't know whether or not God existed, but he was pretty sure He didn't. We were close in childhood, but had let our relationship grow distant as adults. Just after the worst of the worst days back in February when I learned I was likely stage IV, my brother called and asked if there was anything he could do. I replied, "Pray. Please pray for me. I know it doesn't mean much to you, but it means a great deal to me." And he agreed. A few years have passed since then. My brother has prayed for me and he now has come back to a belief in God, though not yet back to Christianity. He's coming back, though. I have faith that he will come back. I have also come to believe that, even in the depths of my own despair, there was something larger going on here. Quite possibly God had a plan for all this suffering I've gone through. I hope so much that this plan includes the conversion of my brother, his wonderful wife and their son. I hope so much that my story will help others come to a better relationship with God. Whatever His plan, I have complete trust that it's a good one.

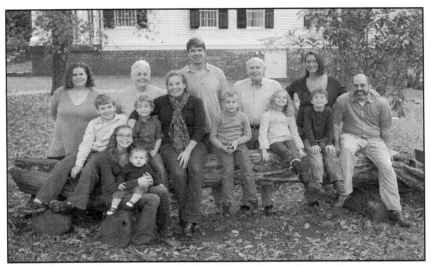

Nicolosi Family

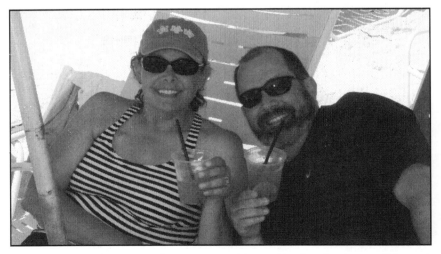

So nice – having cool refreshment with my brother in the Caribbean!

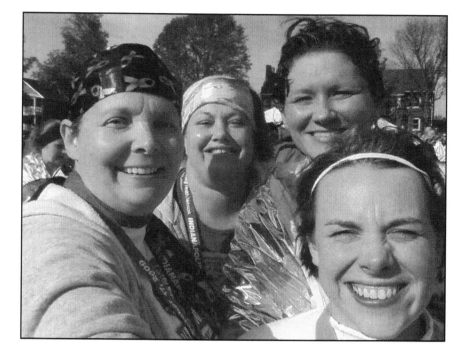

Jen, Christy, Erin and me running for a cure for breast cancer.

getting rid of the buggers

Because we have had our own share of pain, we gain credibility
with those who still suffer. We offer hope in a way that those whose
lives have been untouched by pain cannot. We become living
examples that heartache, broken relationships, physical pain, and
grief are not insurmountable with the help of God.
~ from *Fools, Liars, Cheaters, and Other Bible Heroes*
Barbara Hosbach

The treatment for brain metastases varies depending on
how many there are and how big. Because my mets were dif-
fusely spread throughout my brain, the doctors decided I needed whole brain radiation (the standard care). I was told that
I would lose my hair again and it probably would not grow
back; that I would probably have long term side effects including balance issues, problems with short term memory, and really long term, dementia. As bad as all that sounds, I really had
no other choice and I clung to those words "long term." My
radiation oncologist felt pretty confident that the treatments
would work well to kill off the cancer and that I should be
good for while (at the time, I envisioned years of freedom from
brain mets). Thirteen treatments later, my Caring Bridge entry:

November 22, 2009

God woke me up nice and early this Sunday morning, but it's still a little while until sunrise, so I thought I'd make a quick post. I finished up radiation treatments last Wednesday without having had any real problems. I just get really tired at times and my hair has started to fall out again. Some wonderful friends have gotten quite a collection of new scarves together for me - Rachel and I have had fun trying to put together outfits with them.

We met with both doctors too and both are happy with how I'm doing. I've got my next brain MRI scheduled for December 10th and then we'll review it with Dr. Sapiente on the 14th. It's so nice not to have to go in there for more three weeks!

We are all excited about Thanksgiving around here - Karen and Richard, Steve's parents and brother Dave will be here. We are going to have a wonderful time and I'm so happy we'll be surrounded by family! Cancer has obviously made this year a challenging one, but it hasn't changed the fact that we are also incredibly blessed. Here's my top ten things to be Thankful for this year (well, and always :-)

1. *God's presence in my life - His Peace, Love and Hope*
2. *My husband and children who fill me with joy everyday*
3. *My parents, brother and sister and their families*
4. *Steve's parents and sisters and brothers and their families*
5. *My amazing circle of friends*
6. *My prayer warriors*
7. *Steve's job*
8. *Our house*
9. *All the staff at Carle who've taken such good care of me*
10. *Every single new day.*

I hope you all have a perfectly wonderful Thanksgiving spent with
family and friends and loads of good food –
May God continue to bless each of you!

My next MRI one month later found all but one met had resolved:

Caring Bridge, written Dec 15, 2009 9:20am
Good Morning Everyone! Yesterday's appointment with Dr. Sapi-
ente to review the latest MRI went fairly well, although it was a little
short on useful information. The report was written in such a way
as to confuse not only Steve and I, but Dr. S as well. Overall, things
have improved a lot, and it appears that there is only one tiny spot left.
Dr. S said he is going to get with the Radiologist who read the MRI to
discuss the results and will get back to us. In the mean time, the plan
is that I will have to have additional radiation (targeted this time, and
only 3 rounds) to get rid of it and we are hoping to get that done in the
next couple of weeks...... Yeah, nothing else going on during that time
so it'll be extremely convenient, right :-). Sigh. Well, we have to do
what we have to do. Thankfully, it's only 3 times and the appointments
will be pretty quick - only 30 minutes each. Then maybe I'll have my
unremarkable brain back - I sure hope so!
I have an appointment with Dr. Rowland tomorrow and am hoping
he might have more insight into the MRI reports. And/or we'll get to
talk to Dr. Sapiente again and figure that report out.
Hope you're all enjoying the holiday season - we sure are! We've
been busy, busy but are having fun. The kids are really looking forward
to Christmas break next week and so am I. Grandma and Grandpa
from Florida are coming, as well as my brother and sister and their
families. It may sound like a lot but I will enjoy having my loved ones

so close - I love a loud, family-filled house! Now, if we can just ar-range for some snow for my nephews, it'll be perfect!

There *was* snow that Christmas of 2009; a fact that most might chalk up to simple happenstance, but I say it was Divine Providence. I believe He moves among us and gives us miracle after miracle. We just have to open our eyes of the soul to see. Einstein said "There are two ways to live your life – one is as though nothing is a miracle, the other is as though everything is a miracle." I find myself very much in the latter category. I think the sunrise is a miracle, roses, giraffes, palm trees, stars, crème brulee, a really good red zinfandel and, of course, pup-pies, kittens and babies of all kinds are miracles. I mean, how can you look into the eyes of your children, watch them play, listen to them laugh, see them gently breathe when sleeping against your chest, hear them tell you that they love you and not think "nice job God!" My children are the most magnifi-cent things I have ever beheld and I'm sure I won't ever find anything as amazing in this life, until I get to go Home and see Jesus himself in all His Glory.

My four children have done extremely well throughout this whole ordeal. They amaze me in their resiliency. The young-est two don't really have the understanding that the older two do, but they all know that I am very sick. Thankfully, we have been able to transfer a bit of the old normal into our new normal with relative ease. The beginning of this journey, that whole first year was such a huge roller coaster ride – Disney World, bad news, worse news, Mommy is very sick, Mommy has to go to the hospital every week, Mommy has to nap a lot, Grandma's coming, Grandma's leaving, good news (yay!), summer vacation (yay!), more bad news, Christmas! So much happened that first year and it went by so fast, I feel like cancer stole it from me, especially when it came to my children. We all got a year older, but when I looked at them in February 2010, they had grown so much. How on earth was my baby not a baby anymore, and into the terrible twos?

Caring Bridge, Written Feb 5, 2010 9:51am

Well, today marks my first "cancerversary". It was exactly one year ago today that I got the call from my ob/gyn and she told me the biopsy results came back and that I had cancer. I look back and can just hardly believe it - a year goes by extememly fast. I am very thankful to be feeling pretty good, and able (although it's been a bit challanging lately) to care for my house and family. My energy level is way down from what it used to be though. Aaron, being well into the throes of the terrible twos, has certainly been giving me a run for my money.

To mark the occasion today, I have a doctor's appointment with Dr. Sapiente, a CT scan and an echocardiogram. I think he'll be scheduling my next brain MRI and I'll be getting the results from the other tests next week when I see Dr. Rowland. We are not expecting and changes, but you never know, so please pray things are stable.

This month is going to be just crazy busy and I hope I can keep up. Another benefit to having a new perspective on life is that I am actually looking forward to turning 40 in a week. Not many people can say that :-) Bring on the cake!

That MRI showed that all the cancer had resolved in my brain and a CT scan had shown that the cancer on my liver was stable. I had lost all my hair, the steroids were awful and I puffed up so much as to be nearly unrecognizable, but I was feeling good. Cancer had tried to beat me down, but it didn't and by May 2010, I thought I was winning.

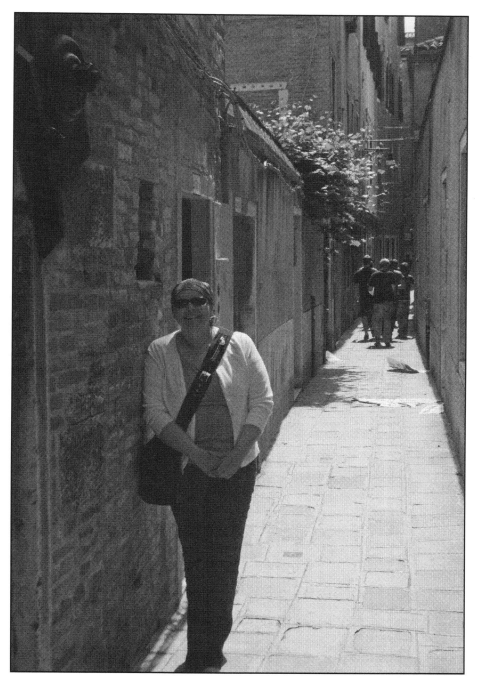

Enjoying time in Italy

travel makes a girl happy

May today there be Peace Within. May you trust that you are exactly where you are meant to be. May you not forget the infinite possibilities that are born of faith in yourself and others. May you use the gifts that you have received, and pass on the love that has been given to you. May you be content with yourself just the way you are. Let this knowledge settle into your bones, and allow your soul the freedom to sing, dance, praise and love.
~ Mother Teresa

To celebrate my first year, Steve and I planned a trip to Italy, another item from the top of my bucket list. We spent ten glorious days there and visited Rome, Florence and Venice. Still on my bucket list, a return trip to Italy to see Assisi, Lake Como, and Tuscany. A girl can dream, right?

We started off our Italian adventure in Rome, the ancient city once at the center of the world and now drenched in Catholicism. Since we are Catholic, this was almost like a homecoming. A lot of other religions have their home bases – this was ours and we felt it. Nuns in habits and Priests in long robes were walking everywhere and on every street corner there appeared another church. Even one of the great ancient roman buildings, the Pantheon, still stands but now is a Catholic church. We went to a lot of them, but by far the most impressive and awe-inspiring was St. Peter's Basilica at the Vatican. Words can't really describe what you feel walking inside – but magnificent and awe-inspiring come close. Off to the right is Michelangelo's Pieta, behind glass now because some idiot tried to shoot at it a little while back. It's stunningly beautiful and though the subject matter is anything but, I distinctly remember feeling at peace looking at it. The whole place was like that, though, once you got past the vastness, even among the throngs of people inside, I felt the wonder of the place. And I felt small. My problems felt small too. It wasn't like all of a sudden I thought my cancer was insignificant, but I was able to put it into perspective. I felt as if God was saying "See, there are bigger things. I am much bigger than you thought." Cancer was not the center of my universe, God was, and is.

Right next door is the Vatican Museum with the Sistine Chapel. You've got to walk past a lot of statues and huge paintings (all beautiful) to get there. It's like when I went to the Louvre in Paris when I was 17, saw lots of stuff (how can I even say that about the vast amount of great art and history on display) on the way to getting to the Mona Lisa. The Mona Lisa was my singular purpose for going to one of the world's finest museums (I was pretty stupid when I was young, I think most of us are). Anyway, even as an adult, I hurried past centuries of great art to get to the reason I came to the Vatican Museum. The Sistine Chapel ceiling is unbelievable and Michelangelo's incredible artistry is beautiful. Unfortunately there were a lot of other admirers in the relatively small space and, though I could have sat and looked at the mastery for hours, I started to feel claustrophobic (which had never happened before chemo/ radiation), and I had to get out of there. But I was so happy to have been there, to have seen something so incredible.

Our next stop was Florence. My father might disinherit me for saying this, but after Rome I was sort of unimpressed... "meh." It's a beautiful city filled with interesting buildings – the Palazzo Vecchio, the Duomo, the Ponte Vecchio, and the great museum Uffizi. What I enjoyed most, though, was the festival going on while we were there. Parades with participants dressed in medieval style and dancing, drum majors marching along; and then there were the Ferraris. They came right along the Arno River and into the Piazza della Signora, hundreds of them from old to brand new. This was a pleasant surprise because we had not heard a thing about the festival before we got there.

And we finished our trip in the lovely, romantic city of Venice. Thankfully we were there before it got hot and so the smell wasn't bad (I had read the warnings). It would have been hard for me to enjoy the city as much if it had smelled like low tide the whole time! But it was wonderful – a city built for walking, and walk we did, and even got lost at one point. Luckily Steve had been to Venice a couple of times before on work trips and sort of knew his way around. I didn't mind getting lost, though. Walking hand in hand with him in that romantic place was sublime. Of course, we had to have a gondola ride which, though expensive and the guy didn't sing, was totally worth it. That evening we went to a 'Violins in Venice' performance at the Chiesa di San Vidal (which, like the festival in Florence, was an unplanned delight) and then Billy Joel walked in with his girlfriend and sat right next to us. Pretty cool! On our last day in Italy we walked to one final church, the Santa Maria della Salute at the very tip of the island of Venice. I felt an incredible sense of peace, something I had not felt in any church save St. Peter's in Rome. As we explored the sanctuary, it was so palpable to me that I mentioned it to Steve. When we came upon a sign that told the story of the church, I couldn't help but smile. Apparently it was built in 1631 after a round of plague had swept throughout the city and a lot of people died. In gratitude for their deliverance, the city built the domed basilica and dedicated it to Our Lady of Health. Cancer felt very far away, but God did not.

Shortly after we returned from Italy, it was time to start planning our annual trip south to visit family. We hadn't made it down the previous year because I was still in the middle of Chemo treatment. We had decided to stay closer to home, but far away enough to call it a vacation, and drove up to Grand Haven, Michigan for a week at a small house right on the lake. Unfortunately, it ended up being the coldest July on record and the week we were there, the temperatures only got to the low 70s. And the water – eek! Was it cold! Anyone who's had chemo knows that cold is a constant state, no matter what. Still, we had a great week at the cabin with fires every night, blueberry picking (lots of pie!) and precious family time.

This year of 2010, after we got to Atlanta, many of our old friends from Georgia Tech wanted to see us. Some good friends volunteered to have a reunion at their house and it was great to see so many of our old gang from college.

The beginning of 2010 turned out pretty great: Cancer mostly gone (WOOT!!!), vacation to Italy (AMAZING!!), trip to Florida (AHHHHH!). Here are some Caring Bridge posts for these events:

Written Apr 9, 2010 9:10am

Great news yesterday! The brain mri shows that all the lesions are gone! I guess my brain will never truly be unremarkable again (due to scar tissue and changes as a result of the radiation), but this is pretty darn close. Now, we just need to keep it that way :) I know you all were praying for this result - thank you! God does hear our prayers!

Coming up next: I will probably have a bone scan next week - my back has been bothering me for the last few weeks and hasn't really gotten better. The nurse thinks it's another side effect of one of the drugs I'm on (Tykerb), but we're doing the scan to make sure. I'll be getting treatment next week and then my next appointment is with Dr. Rowland at the end of this month.

We are enjoying this beautiful spring sunshine and hope you are too. We've got lots to do this weekend - fun stuff like washing the car, cleaning out the garage and mowing the grass, but it'll be great just to be outside. We're also planning Katherine's birthday party - 14 five year old girls.... should be lots of fun (and loud :-). And finally, Steve and I are making our final travel plans for Italy. Can't wait!!!

Hope your weekend is as fun-filled!

Written May 24, 2010 1:43pm

Just a quick update today. We had an appointment last Wednesday with Dr. Rowland and everything looks good. The only thing he was even remotely worried about was that my red blood cell count is a little low. Hopefully it's nothing some iron pills and a few steaks won't take care of :)

We had a fantastic trip to Italy, but it was good to get back home to the kiddos. My favorite place was Rome, followed by a close second, Venice. Everything we saw was just jaw-dropping. I really like history so to stand and walk around in places that are 2000 years old was really cool. Now, we've gotten back into the swing of things and I think I may finally be over my jet lag! I'll post some pictures soon.

Laura Dahl

I also wanted to invite all of you to help me raise money for the American Cancer Society. I will be participating in the Relay for Life on June 12th for my good friend Jesse's team. If you'd like to make a donation, please follow this link to my ACS Relay for Life page (you may have to copy it and paste into your address line):

https://secure3.convio.net/tacs/site/Donation2?idb=906565088&df_id=1007667&FR_ID=22121&PROXY_ID=16648445&PROXY_TYPE=20&1007667.donation=form1

Thanks so much for all your support. Life is Good!

Written Aug 3, 2010 8:30am

Hope everyone is having a wonderful summer - we are! I can't believe it's been such a long time since I last posted, but as they say, no news is good news (for now at least!). I have been feeling very well for the past couple of months, and although those headaches are still around, they are mild and haven't gotten worse. Other than that, things are great!

We have had a pretty busy summer so far, but now are in the home stretch and getting ready for school to start back up again (which the older two are not happy about, but the younger two make up for their lack of enthusiasm with bounds of excitement). Our trip down south to Atlanta and Florida was so much fun. We got to see lots of friends and family that we hadn't seen in many years - it was so great to see everyone and catch up. Thanks again to our dear friends Scott and Gina for hosting our GT reunion! After all the fun in Atlanta, we headed further south to stay with my parents in Florida. Loved, loved, LOVED that Florida sunshine! My brother and sister and their families came by too, so it was lots of fun. I got to see my dear Aunt, who also has breast cancer - love you Aunt Karen!

To top all that off, my friend Christy and I flew out to Las Vegas for a "Mom's weekend off". We had such a great time and saw two fabulous shows - Cirque du Soleil "the Beatles Love" and Jerry Sein-feld Live. We lost some money, but had a lot of fun anyway! We both agreed that next time we need to stay at least a day or two longer!

I'm still getting treatment every 3 weeks and a shot every four weeks, but Dr. Rowland has moved his appointments to every 8 weeks. I will be going back to see him again on Aug. 25th. I am so thankful for each and every day, and for feeling as well as I do. I am so thankful for my beautiful family and for all of you. Please keep us in your prayers and pray for a cure.

Enjoy these waning days of summer - they're going to go by fast!

Written Aug 31, 2010 8:49am

What a great summer we have had! The kids have started back to school and we're all getting back into the swing of things. I had a Dr.'s appointment last Wednesday and things are still looking good. I don't see him again until Nov. 3rd and he will probably order a scan at that time just to check things out - the last one was about 6 months ago!

I have felt very good all summer - pretty much back to normal - and it's been wonderful. I am so thankful to be able to take care of the kids and do things I used to do. It's a good thing too - it seems like our schedules just exploded since school started! Life is full speed ahead for us - just the way I like it.

Have a great Labor Day weekend!

Up until November of 2010, things were really looking great and we were able to have so much fun! I know those months were a great gift from God after such a hard year before. Reading through my journal entries for 2010 revealed to me how good that year really was. Things changed of course, but I thank God so very much for the time to enjoy my family and feel His Love surrounding us.

Laura Dahl

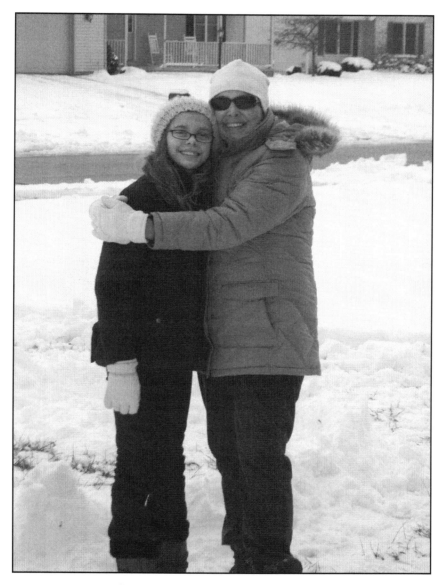

Me and my beautiful oldest – I love you Rachel!
(Love snow? Eh, not so much.)

trouble sneaks back

And the God of all grace, who called you to his eternal glory in
Christ, after you have suffered a little while, will himself restore you
and make you strong, firm and steadfast.

~ 1 Peter 5:10

Well, not all of November 2010 was bad. I had a PET Scan
which showed amazing results. Here's what the bottom of the
doctor's report said (emphasis added by me!):

IMPRESSION: Marked interval response. **Clearing of
previously described metastatic areas of
involvement since 2009 study.**

Love, love, love that word "clearing!" This meant that all of
the previous cancer below my neck was resolved, taken care
of, finished, spent, depleted, GONE! What amazing news and I
thought that I was in the clear.

The MRI however, was completely different. I don't even

know how to begin. Ugh.

In the beginning of December, I had another MRI after the fantastic PET scan to see how things were going in the brain, which had been going very well all year. I had been treated with the whole brain radiation at the end of the previous year (2009) and had been doing really well with that plus Herceptin and Tykerb. And though I was starting to have some headaches, I was still hopeful they were nothing related to the cancer. I was wrong. Here's the Caring Bridge report from December 4, 2010:

Written Dec 4, 2010 9:36am

One of the hardest things about life with cancer is the extremes. One day you're riding high from a great PET scan result, and the next, trying to cope with a dismal MRI result. Dr. Rowland called me (I knew THAT was not a good sign) yesterday evening with the bad news. I have a 1.1cm tumor near my cerebellum, very close to or at the spot of the tumor they zapped in January. There are other spots that are "suspicious". He has already discussed my case with radiation oncology and they don't think that's an option because that spot has already received radiation. He was going to talk to the neurosurgeons about surgical options, either here at Carle or down at Barnes in St. Louis. We have an appointment with him on Monday to develop a plan.

As I walked out of the Cancer Center yesterday after my MRI, I was feeling so good, so confident. Today, I am just trying to make sure to breathe regularly and not break down in front of the children. This is so unfair for them. I am trying not to be crushed by this news, but it is difficult.

Lord, help me to climb out of the clutches of despair. Help me to see your light always shining in front of me. Help me to know you are with me at all times. Help Steve and the children know you are with them at all times. Lord, bring us your Peace.

Amen

With that comment that afternoon though, the next day was so much better. God has an amazing way of resetting my heart and soul. This is one of my very favorite posts and I felt such peace that morning, I knew I had to say something.

Written Dec 5, 2010 10:00am

After yesterday's depressing entry, and with how I feel this morning, I thought I had better post again. Today I feel so much better. I have had an epiphany of sorts - as the old saying goes "Today is the first day of the rest of your life." Cancer has taken so much time away from me already, and I'll be d@*ned if I'm going to let it take one more second because I am sad or wallowing in self-pity. No, I will not let that happen any more. Life is too short and the joys therein too precious. I feel very much at peace this morning and I trust God completely with my life. It's been His all along anyway. I hope I can convey these truths to my children and that they find comfort in them. I know I do.

Have a wonderful Sunday! We will be enjoying the 8 inches of snow we got yesterday and tonight we'll be back at church for the Advent Celebration!

God clearly knew I needed a lift, and boy is He so good at that! My next entry though, the next day, was miserable. "Ugly" I called it. The brain mets had mostly returned, but still pretty small with the largest one measuring 1.1 cm and other small ones throughout the brain and the cerebellum. Not good. Dr. Sapiente was not happy and had quite a negative treatment outlook. We talked to a neurosurgeon at Carle to find out if there were any options in that area. We were told by the very nice doctor that he really couldn't do anything because there were so many lesions all over my brain, too many to remove with surgery. We decided to go back to St. Louis and talk to them about options, which essentially included more radiation. After all I had heard and read and experienced, I wasn't exactly thrilled about that option. All in all, it was pretty easy to feel depressed again, but there was one more card I was holding.

Drs. Rowland and Sapiente recommended I go out to Dana Farber in Boston to seek a third opinion. They had apparently been working on breast cancer brain mets for a while and were getting ready to introduce a new phase 2 trial. I had read a little about the doctor there and how much he was doing because the Her2 brain mets were becoming more of a problem with Herceptin. Herceptin is a fantastic drug, really a miracle, but it seems clear now that it has trouble getting into the brain to fight off the tumors there. The molecules are too big to penetrate the blood brain barrier. From John's Hopkins:

"The blood-brain barrier is a dynamic interface that separates the brain from the circulatory system and protects the central nervous system from potentially harmful chemicals while, at the same time, regulating transport of essential molecules and maintaining a stable environment," Searson said. "It is formed from highly specialized endothelial cells that line the brain capillaries, which transduce signals in two directions: from the vascular system and from the brain. The structure and function of the BBB is dependent upon the complex interplay between different cell types, specifically the endothelial cells, astrocytes and pericytes, within the extracellular matrix of the brain and with the blood flow in the capillaries."

Although the BBB serves the important purpose of tightly regulating the environment of the brain and preventing sudden changes, which the brain cannot tolerate, Searson said, "this interface also blocks the passage of drug molecules to treat disease, neurodegenerative disorders, inflammation or stroke. Unfortunately, animal models are insufficient for use in understanding how the human blood-brain barrier functions or responds to drugs. In addition, little is known about how disease, inflammation or stroke disrupts or damages the blood-brain barrier."

Dr. Rowland suggested we head out to Dana Farber as soon as possible and discuss treatment options they could offer. This trip ended up being a miracle, complete with knowledge God was watching us.

Caring Bridge, Written Jan 17, 2011 8:11am

Thank you all so much for the safe and successful travel prayers - we had a fantastic trip to Boston! Last Tuesday, I was really wondering if it would even happen, what with Atlanta being shut down for days and the epic nor'east-er headed right toward Boston. God was watching out for us though - while most of Atlanta was still snow and ice-bound, the airport had opened 4 of 5 runways and our flight into Atlanta was on-time (this is amazing even without considering the city had been shut down, it's the busiest airport in the world). What I was really concerned about was our flight to Hartford (we were flying there instead of Boston to see our dear friends the Paulsons). Delta had cancelled 4 of 6 flights to Hartford Wednesday morning and by the time we got on our flight that afternoon, the pilot informed us that it was the only one not cancelled. And it was on time. When we landed, the airport was actually closed because 20 inches of snow had fallen

Laura Dahl

that day - we didn't even have to circle the airport to give the ground crew time to plow again (they were out in force though, the runways were pretty clear). Not only was our flight on-time (which, how often is Delta on-time now a days anyway?), but Karen's flight from Chicago landed safely and on-time an hour and a half behind ours (it was still snowing and the airport was still officially closed). Divine Providence at work is awesome!

Our appointments at Dana Farber went extremely well. The doctors were very nice, and more importantly, very informed and each spent at least an hour with us. They both specialize in brain metastases and we got excellent advice - we now have a plan. In fact, the medical oncologist has already talked to Dr. Rowland about her recommendations. First thing on our plan is to have another MRI to establish a baseline. If nothing has changed, or if the tumors are smaller (please God!), we keep on the chemo that I'm currently on. If they have increased in size or number, we go to a new chemo combo that has been proven in studies to reach the brain pretty well. In about 4 months, the doctor we saw will be starting a clinical trial of a new drug that looks promising and she said I would qualify for it. Down the road a ways (hopefully, a long ways!) I could look at joining this trial. The only thing is that it will be run out of Boston and would require monthly trips there. But we'll cross that bridge when we come to it.

The radiation oncologist we met with told us about the options that area could provide. Because I'm not really having any symptoms, she recommended going the chemo route first and delaying radiation for as long as possible. I'm good with that :)

Finally, we thoroughly enjoyed visiting with our friends. Fabulous meals and desserts (as expected ;), cards (girls win! I warned you Mike ;), and spending time with some of the cutest kids ever. Loved it - thank you all so much for a wonderful visit!

I am not sure when the MRI will be, but I really hope it's sometime this week - we've delayed long enough. I'll try to post something when I know. Prayers are always welcome and accepted :-)

http://www.dana-farber.org/Adult-Care/Treatment-and-Support/ Brain-Metastasis.aspx

During this first trip, it was decided that the new drug, Neratinib, they were working on getting to trial would be their recommendation. Unfortunately, it wasn't yet through Dana Farber's approval process. Dr. Freedman gave me an estimate of the late spring for it to be available (in actuality, it wasn't available until December 2011). She recommended that I stay on my current drugs for as long as possible.

Soon after I returned to Carle, we got some highly desired good news!

Caring Bridge - Written Jan 22, 2011 8:48am

Living with cancer really is like living on a roller coaster, with all the highs and lows and turns - sometimes it's hard to hold on. The MRI results were surprisingly good - I say that because I honestly thought they would show slight progression. But, when I talked to my nurse on Thursday, she read the last part of the report to me - all I remember were the words "stable" and "decreased". When we met with Dr. Rowland we got to read the report and look at the images. Here's the gist of it:

1. Stable small metastases in cerebellum, precuneus and parahippocampal gyrus (yeah, I have no idea either - stable is the important word there)

2. Decreased size of right temporal metastasis and resolution of bi-

Laura Dahl

lateral cerebellar metastases. No new lesions.

Also noteworthy is that the lesions that were on my skull have completely resolved.

I like the way this guy talks! I really didn't think there would be improvement because the only change we made to my treatment was to increase the dose of one of the drugs (Tykerb) I had already been on for a year. Obviously the reduced dose (750mg) wasn't doing anything for me as the brain mets popped up anyway. It's remarkable that going up 500 more mg has helped so dramatically in such a relatively short period of time (about 4 weeks).

So the plan is to continue with my current regimen and to get another MRI in 6 weeks. I'll also have to get another echocardiagram next month to check heart function. We can celebrate for now, but my situation is still quite "serious" - in the immortal words of Han Solo, "Don't get cocky, kid". We may not be able to be cocky about the cancer, but we can be utterly confident in God's plan whatever course this disease takes. Thanks so much for keeping up with the ride and for your continued prayers!

In March 2011, I dropped Herceptin and added Zeloda. May 2011 brought good news again:

Caring Bridge, Written May 4, 2011 2:39pm

Another beautiful sunny day, and a day to rejoice in the goodness of God. I had my MRI this morning and saw Dr. Rowland this afternoon - the news was very encouraging! The three largest lesions have decreased in size and the multiple new lesions that showed up on the last MRI have either "significantly decreased in size or have completely resolved" YAY - the new drug is working! So we will march on with my current regimen and continue to pray it works :) Next MRI will be scheduled for 8 weeks unless I start to have symptoms before then.

Now we can really celebrate when we go on our Disney cruise vacation - and I guarantee we will! Thanks again for the support and prayers - I will be toasting to all of you!

I also wanted to mention that I am participating in the American Cancer Society's Relay for Life again this year. Last year, I think I raised something like $900. This year I'd like to raise $1000. You can visit my fund-raising web page here:

http://main.acsevents.org/site/TR?fr_id=30563&pg=entry

Thank you so much!

"The Lord bless you and keep you;

The Lord make His face shine upon you,

And be gracious to you; The Lord look upon you kindly, and give you Peace!

Numbers 6:24-26

Laura Dahl

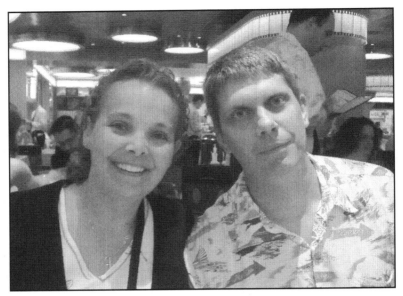

On the Disney Cruise with Steve!

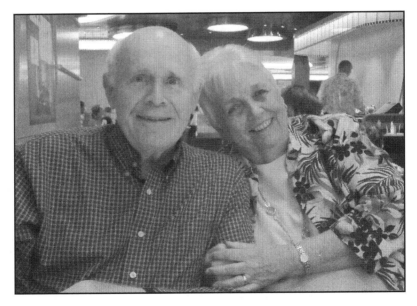

Dad and Mom, cruising with us.

Disney Cruise

All our dreams can come true
if we have the courage to pursue them.
~ Walt Disney

"Well, I brought this book on vacation with every intention of writing every day. And the whole thing just blew by without a single word. We truly had an absolutely wonderful, perfectly magical time. It seems almost like a dream (pun intended)."

That was the first paragraph of my diary entry on May 22, 2011. I wrote about the whole trip (good job me!) and it's filled with great memories. I choose to include some of what I wrote here because we had such a fun, care-free time and the cancer problem seemed to step back for us and there's no medical reference here at all. It was just a fantastic vacation. Here are some entries I chose because each experience I was writing about was in some way special.

Laura Dahl

Day 1 – Magic Kingdom. "Our first day was jam-packed with fun at the Magic Kingdom. First ride was the Jungle Cruise and Aaron got to be Captain! Then off to Pirates of the Caribbean – my favorite! And a show right outside the ride. Aaron got a starring role in this as well – and got to meet Captain Jack Sparrow himself!"

Day 2 - Boarding the ship. We explored the ship –found the Oceaneer's Club, the Edge, the pools, the AquaDuck, and were amazed! Mom, Dad, Mandy, Joe and Alex and the kids all went to dinner at the Royal Palace while Steve and I joined Karen and Richard at Remy. What an experience – hands down the best dining experience I'd ever had! We were there for 3 hours! Something like six courses and all were amazing food with hand-selected wine by the sommelier, and incredible service. It was without doubt the best dinner I have ever had.

Day 3 – At Nassau. We disembarked midmorning and went to the Pirate Museum. Thank goodness we had Joe for a guide – he knew exactly where to go. A guy was there dressed up as a pirate and the kids had fun giving him a hard time. The museum was small but interesting and the gift shop was a 3-year-old pirate lover's dream."

Day 4 – At Castaway Cay. Castaway Cay is beautiful and well designed by Disney to handle a large crowd…Snorkeling was disappointing because there wasn't much to see (except jellyfish, one of which decided I was too close and stung me)! Rachel and Ben enjoyed the experience, though Ben more than Rachel. I had a really good time on the beach and Disney did a good job of providing lots of adult frozen drinks! Joe and I had a great time playing with Katherine, Aaron and Alex on the beach and in the shallow water. We hardly saw Karen and Richard, but I can't blame them for finding some quieter space!

Later that evening we went up to deck 11 for the fireworks show, which was "Pirates of the Caribbean" themed (shocking!) It was pretty silly, but the fireworks were great, and then a dance party. Whew, were we tired by the end of the day!

Day 5 – At Sea. This was one of my favorite days – relaxing. After breakfast, everyone scattered. Rachel and I walked around the ship (wish we'd played shuffleboard)! Katherine and Aaron went to the Oceaneer's Club. Ben and Steve checked out the arcade. After lunch, Mom, Mandy and I went to the wine tasting … (and) after we got on our swimsuits and headed to the pool. Mom and I went on the Aqua Duck – very happy she went out of her comfort zone and went on it! Dinner at Palo with Karen and Richard as delicious, but not as good as Remy – but I guess no restaurant can top Remy! It was a really good day and since we knew we were leaving early the next morning we knew we had to take advantage of as many things as we could squeeze in!

Day 6 – Disembarkation. Had to wake up very early (I think it was 5:30 a.m.) and had breakfast at Enchanted Garden and said goodbye to our service team. Vanya and the others were so good to us. We disembarked and said good bye to Karen and Richard so they could catch their flight back home. We drove off to Orlando and met Sarah, Justin and little Logan. All the kids had a great time playing at the pool and then went to Downtown Disney for dinner at T Rex. It's a great blessing from God that both my family and Steve's get along so well!

Caring Bridge, Written Jun 29, 2011 8:05pm

More praise for our wonderful God - plan B is still working! Had my scans last Friday and reviewed them with Dr. Rowland today. PET scan shows no disease in soft tissue and the spine mets have improved. Brain MRI shows, that of the three tumors present on the last scan (8

Laura Dahl

weeks ago) , one is relatively stable, one has decreased in size, and the third has resolved. At the appointment today, Dr. R was downright happy - and for an oncologist, that's saying something. As you can probably imagine, good news appointments are so much nicer than bad news. We didn't even discuss when my next appointment will be or when the next scans will be - I love walkin' out of there with a smile on my face :)

We will be leaving soon for our trip south to visit family and friends. Atlanta for the 4th and then on to Florida to see the Space Shuttle launch and lots of fun in the sun! We are very much looking forward to seeing everyone and celebrating!

I wish I could attach music to this post - if I could it would be "Walking on Sunshine" by Katrina and the Waves. Such a great, feel-good, happy song. That's how I'm am right now - feeling great and very happy and thankful to be alive. Too many blessings to count, and thankful for every single one of them.

"I will praise you, Lord, with all my heart; I will declare all your wondrous deeds. I will delight and rejoice in you; I will sing hymns to your name, Most High. For my enemies turn back; they stumble and perish before you." Psalm 9:2-4

"I trust in your faithfulness. Grant my heart joy in your help, that I may sing of the Lord, 'How good our God has been to me!'" Psalm 13:6

October 2011 – The Good Stuff Just Doesn't Last …

Caring Bridge, Written Oct 19, 2011 6:22pm
Well folks, I wish I had better news to share on this very dreary day. My brain MRI showed that the cancer is progressing - not only have the previous ones grown, but there are a couple of new ones. They're still all pretty small, thank goodness. But still. It sucks. I

did get some good news though - the PET scan showed that, below the neck, there is no evidence of disease.

So now we have to come up with Plan C. Unfortunately, I don't think that the clinical trial out in Boston is up and running yet. We're still going to fly out there to talk to them about other options though. We may even head back down to St. Louis to get their opinion. I need as much advice as I can get - kinda stuck between a rock and hard place right now.

I'm sure many of you know of the Tim McGraw song "Live Like You Were Dying". I heard it on the radio Monday on my way home from the scans (and I hadn't heard it in probably 5 years or so) and I thought to myself, "yep that's what I'm doing". Well, no skydiving for me, but living with a life-threatening illness puts everything into very clear perspective. Prioritizing things in your life becomes extremely easy. My faith, my family, my friends are everything to me.

"I went sky diving, I went rocky mountain climbing,
I went two point seven seconds on a bull named Fu Man Chu.
And I loved deeper and I spoke sweeter,
And I gave forgiveness I'd been denying.
An' he said: "Some day, I hope you get the chance,
To live like you were dyin'."
Like tomorrow was a gift,
And you got eternity,
To think about what you'd do with it.
An' what did you do with it?
An' what can I do with it?
An' what would I do with it?"

Tomorrow is indeed a gift and I intend to make the most of it :)
Love to you all! ~Laura

Laura Dahl

November 2011 – it's back to real life and on to Boston.

Caring Bridge, Written Nov 12, 2011 1:31pm

We're back from a great and fruitful trip out to Boston. If you're ever in Boston, I can highly recommend The Beehive restaurant. The food and service were fantastic, but I must admit that it was the company we were with that made it even better. Thanks so much to our dear friends Mike and Beth for driving out (through the downpour and traffic!) to meet us, for staying up late visiting, and for buying dinner (we get the next one though!). And am also so thankful for my wonderful sister-in-law Karen who flew in Friday morning to be with us for our appointment. I love you guys!

I really like both doctors we saw at Dana Farber/Brigham & Women's. They both spent a lot of time with us and let us ask as many questions as we could think of and didn't rush us at all. We have a very clear picture of what's going on inside this noggin of mine. The Radiation Oncologist reviewed all of my MRI's from this year and compared them to the ones I had back in 2009. She spent a good amount of time explaining her recommendation (including the risks) and, whereas before I was really hesitant to do any more radiation therapy, now I feel much more comfortable with the idea.

The Medical Oncologist was so great - not only is she a talented, highly intelligent doctor, she's extremely personable and easy to talk to. She also gave us as much time as we needed to ask questions and explained her recommendations thoroughly. She agrees with her colleague, that I should have targeted radiation on the two most prominent tumors and take a chemo holiday and change back to Herceptin only (which will be so nice because Herceptin has very few side effects). The really good news is that the clinical trial she spoke to me about last time looks like it's finally going to open by January. And in addition to that trial, there's another one coming shortly after that features a new drug which specifically targets Her2 positive breast cancer brain metastases. Woot! - finally, some seriously good options! I meet with Dr. Rowland this Wednesday to discuss these recommendations and make a plan.

I also have to give very special thanks to two truly great friends, Diane and Christy, who took care of our kids for us while we were gone. You both are such a blessing, not only to me, but to my family as well. I love you two! And for all my other friends and family that supported me in prayer, and continue to do so, thank you so much, I love you all too!

Saw this poem painted on the wall in the walkway between Dana Farber and Brigham and Women's, loved it and actually remembered who it was by:

Hope is the Thing With Feathers

Hope is the thing with feathers
That perches in the soul,
And sings the tune without the words,
And never stops at all,
And sweetest in the gale is heard;
And sore must be the storm
That could abash the little bird
That kept so many warm.
I've heard it in the chillest land,
And on the strangest sea;
Yet, never, in extremity,
It asked a crumb of me.
- Emily Dickinson

Laura Dahl

Thankful

Caring Bridge, Written Nov 23, 2011 7:36am

I realize this is an obvious statement, but sometimes life is hard - I think God designed it that way to give us even more opportunities to overcome challenges and to love others. And of course, to become even closer to Him. I am thankful for so very many things that it would be practically impossible to list them all. Back in summer of 2009, right in the middle of chemo, we took a vacation to Grand Haven, MI and the house we rented was right on Lake Michigan – the sunsets were magnificent. I said out loud many times that "life is good" and it's kind of been my mantra ever since. I think it's a great gift to be able to say this, and for that, I'm thankful too.

So, since my last post I have seen my local doctors and they both agree with the doctors out east (another answered prayer – consensus). Next week, I will have a "thin-slice" MRI and get a mask made for radiation treatment. They will have to plan how to get to the mets, but I'm hopeful to get the treatments early to mid December. I'll keep you posted :)

Surrounded by family and friends, tons of food, and lots of laughter, I hope you all have a fantastic Thanksgiving weekend!

"Be joyful always; pray continually; give thanks in all circumstances, for this is God's will for you in Christ Jesus." 1 Thessalonians 5: 16-18

Shine

Caring Bridge, Written Dec 2, 2011 8:20am

Okay, things are going faster than I thought they would – which is good because this month is going to be crazy enough! This week, I had a long (very long!) MRI which showed that there weren't any more little buggers hiding out anywhere. Then, I was fitted for my mask, which they use to keep my head very still. So I will start the first of five radiation treatments on Monday and then everyday next week. I have to go back on steroids (blech!) so if I look like I've gained fifty pounds, it's not due to over-indulging this holiday season (well, I will just a little). I hope to only be on them for a week or two, so maybe I won't get as puffy as last time.

I've been asked by several people this past month if I feel that I am inspirational (which is kinda weird for so many in such a short period of time). And at first I thought well, I don't know (and my humility warning bells went off) - how would I know that? Then the answer came to me, "I hope so". I don't mean to get preachy, but I think this is important: One of the things I believe we are supposed to do as Christians is to reflect the Light and Love of Christ to everyone we know and love, and to everyone we meet. We should shine for Him. I certainly don't do it all the time, but I pray constantly for the strength to, and when I fail (which happens almost daily - I am a work in progress:) I ask for forgiveness.

This song is exactly what I'm talking about: Shine, by Salvador:

"Lord let me shine, shine like the moon, a reflection of You, in all that I do. Let me be a light for Your Truth. Light of the world, I wanna be used to shine for You."

I'll post again sometime after treatments and hopefully before Christmas. Enjoy the season, and remember the reason :)

So in December I had to get additional radiation treatments for the remaining 4 tumors. We had a wonderful Christmas, with a visit from my brother Joe and his family, Mandy and little Alex.

By the end of January 2012 my brain mets seemed to be resolving and overall, things were looking good. As you've noticed throughout this book, my process with cancer has had a lot of ups and downs. Of course all our lives are like that to a degree, it's just that having a life-threatening disease makes the roller coaster-like falls seem even greater. Two months later the cancer really hadn't gone anywhere. Thank goodness we had a good plan to go to next – Dana Farber.

Sigh....

But my next entry –

Life is Good
Caring Bridge, Written Apr 18, 2012 9:30am

I just wanted to post a quick update. I have gotten all my appointments at Dana Farber to start the clinical trial. Still working on the logistics of getting and staying there, but they're coming along too. It's such a blessing to have that in progress and has eased my anxiety considerably. I'll go through the whole gamut of tests and if I still qualify for the trial after all that, I will start Friday May 4th - WOOT!

I have been very busy working on the Cursillo team I am leading. It's been a huge blessing in my life working with these ladies who are just incredible and are such strong witnesses for Christ. I am thankful beyond words and so inspired - it's gonna be an amazing weekend! Please pray for us and the candidates who will be going through.

It's going to be a beautiful day here in central Illinois and I plan to enjoy it. I've got flowers to plant and weeds to pull. :)

"A joyful heart is like the sunshine of God's Love, the hope of eternal happiness, a burning flame of God. And if we pray, we will become that sunshine of God's Love - in our home, the place where we

live and in the world at large." ~Mother Teresa

This is another example of how Cursillo has changed my life and has brought me more of God's grace than I could possibly begin to understand and appreciate enough.

Laura Dahl

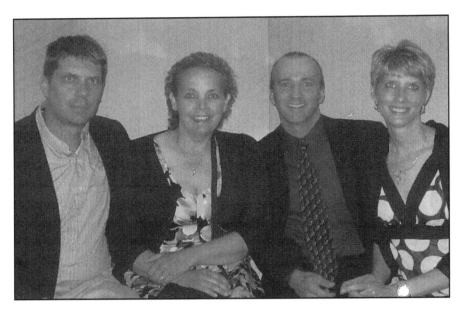

Best meal at Disney, made even better by sharing it with
Karen and Richard.

Boston Marathon
my own

My brothers and sisters, whenever you face trials of any kind,
consider it nothing but joy, because you know that the testing
of your faith produces endurance; and let endurance have its
full effect, so that you may be mature and complete,
lacking in nothing.

~ James 1:2-4

Boston is a great city and despite the reason for the visits, I fell for it hook, line and sinker. I don't remember any part that I didn't like. Well, maybe the snow that first visit. But I think it's one of the best cities I've had the privilege of visiting. And staying with Mandy's Aunt Betsy and her husband, Bill, in Watertown was a huge blessing. There is so much to see and investigate – I loved going on Harvard campus, Chinatown, the Red Sox games, the restaurants, the subway was even interesting to me!

I started the trial treatment in May and things went well to begin with. Dana Farber is very near the center of Boston and thanks to our friends, getting there on the T from Watertown (which was about 5 miles away as the crow flies, but 30 minutes on the bus and train) was pretty easy.

Laura Dahl

The good, the bad, and the wonderful
Caring Bridge, Written May 5, 2012 8:12am

First, the good. Everything went pretty well at Dana Farber – spent all day there on Wednesday and most of the day there on Thursday getting a thorough screening. Blood work, urinalysis, MRI, CTscan, bone scan, and on Friday a neurocognitive exam, which thankfully didn't involve math. The cancer is still in remission form the neck down (WOOT!) – the cancer is obviously still in my brain because I am on the clinical trial. But I am very optimistic about this drug – we were told that of the patients already on the trial (since January) all had shown good results on the drug – very encouraging!

The bad. The weather was pretty awful the entire time we were there – 40's and rainy. Which would be perfectly fine when you can stay at home snuggled up with a good book. Not so much when you're walking to bus stations and to the hospital from the train station or while sitting at a Red Sox game. But there was lots of good even through this - we had no problems navigating the T and the game was lots of fun, despite the loss and the cold. I was just so happy to be at Fenway and seeing a MLB game (it had been probably been about 12 years since I went to one).

The wonderful. We got to stay with some pretty great people this trip. My sister-in-law Mandy hooked us up with her Aunt and Uncle who live just outside of Boston, about 5 miles away, and just a few steps away from the bus line that took us to the T. Though it took a while to get to the hospital, it was very convenient. We were shown every courtesy and kindness and the house was beautiful. Thank you so much Betsy and Bill! And I want to say a very special thank you for my wonderful sister-in-law Karen, who has been such a fantastic support for me and Steve, who made the trip out with me. Love you Karen!

I'll be back in Boston every 4 weeks, so I will try to post after I get back each time. The big news will come in 8 weeks after I get another MRI and we can see what effect the drug is having.

Lots of Hope, lots of Peace, and lots of Love!

~Laura

Things at Dana Farber continued to go well. Another Red Sox game – this time with Steve and me both nice and warm in the summer time. Oh yeah, the tickets were a gift and in the 6th row behind the batter's box. Amazing! Thanks so much to a friend of Steve's who has other connected and substantial friends wanting to help too!

Noticeable improvement – Woot!

Caring Bridge, Written Jun 30, 2012 1:51pm

The trip to Boston was a complete success (well, except for my overconfidence in knowing the T) - the preliminary MRI results show "noticeable improvement." I will get the final report late next week, but Dr. F was very happy with the results, which of course, makes me happy! My CT continues to show that things below the neck are "unremarkable" (such a wonderful word) and my echocardiogram and blood work came back normal.

Steve went with me this trip, mostly because getting results can be either one of two things, joyous or crushing, and at these appointments it's really a good idea to have a loved one with you (either to celebrate with or to hold on to). I wanted him to be with me for these first results and he wanted to be there too. Because of some scheduling issues, we got to be in Boston a day and a half early and just have some fun. We had some great dinners with friends (nice seeing you again Charlie and meeting your lovely wife Anita; and Mike and Beth – it was wonderful, as always, seeing you again!) and went to an afternoon

Red Sox game (great seats and they won!) and got to see some sights (some on purpose, some accidental).

We had a fantastic trip out west earlier this month too. I'll try to post some pictures, but it's impossible to capture the splendor and wonder of what we saw. We went to Grand Canyon, Arches, Bryce Canyon and Zion National Parks and drove through 1500 miles of some of the most unique and amazing lands I have ever seen. It was beauty and grandeur and awe all rolled up together.

Never lose an opportunity for seeing anything that is beautiful; For beauty is God's handwriting – a wayside sacrament. Welcome it in every fair face, in every fair sky, in every fair flower, And thank God for it as a cup of His blessing.
- Ralph Waldo Emerson

That cup runneth over in my case. Many, many blessings!

Peace,
Laura

P.S. I almost forgot – please, please pray for a stage 4 friend of mine, Jen, who recently found out that her cancer is advancing. She is an inspiration to me and everyone she knows and loves. Please pray that she and her doctors can find a clinical trial that will work miracles for her. And pray for her son (age 5) and family too. God bless you, Jen!

Jen ended up passing in the fall 2013. I was so sad. And the news seemed so unbelievable. She was a beautiful friend filled with so much knowledge. I am so blessed to have known her – she will be incredibly missed.

bucket list trips continue

And the God of all grace, who called you to his eternal glory
in Christ, after you have suffered a little while, will himself
restore you and make you strong, firm and steadfast.
~ 1 Peter 5:10

Of course, we had to go somewhere on vacation that summer and get that bucket list attended to ... even during treatment, vacations and time spent with family are crucial. As I briefly mentioned in a Caring Bridge note above, we had an amazing trip out west in June. Our first stop, simply because the flights made sense, was Las Vegas. If you're wondering why we would take the kids there, well, looking back, you're thinking along the same lines I am. This wasn't really part of the vacation, just the closest place we could fly into, and we decided we'd only stay the day then drive on to the Hoover Dam and then the Grand Canyon. Katherine, being an extremely observant seven year-old, had lots to say – primarily about how "inappropriate" the whole town was. Every time she saw an ad with a half naked

Laura Dahl

person on it, God bless her, she'd say "Mommy, everything here is so inappropriate! I can't look anywhere!" We decided then and there that was our last stay in Vegas. We left the next day for the prime destination of our trip – The Grand Canyon – but made another little stop, this time at Hoover Dam. We mostly enjoyed it, but Rachel had no interest at all and wasn't afraid to express her disapproval. For those of you with young teen agers, you know they can make a trip completely "un-fun." Luckily for her, and for us, we only stayed a few hours and started the drive out to Arizona.

I was so looking forward to the Grand Canyon, but I also knew it was a bit of a drive to get there from Vegas, about four hours. As always, I discovered the journey there had a silver lining. Granted, there was a ton of, well nothing but brush, but we also got to see spectacular rock formations out in the fields. Huge! And we recognized a lot from movies we'd seen – so fun! When we finally arrived, it was getting late so we decided we'd go to the park in the morning. Mandy and Joe didn't want to wait. They wanted to go see the canyon at sunrise, which that far west was at about 5 a.m. After they left, I realized that I really wanted to see it for the first time then too. As it turned out, none of the other adults wanted to go or they were still asleep, so I hopped into the rental and drove out to the rim about two miles north of where we were staying. After I got there I just walked north until the edge found me and then my breath was literally taken away. I immediately fell into prayer because I was getting a glimpse of God and He is magnificent … really amazing! I am so unbelievably happy God called me to see that and I will carry the image in me from now on.

While we were still in Arizona, we went down to Sedona and got some tourist shopping in. The landscape was beauti-

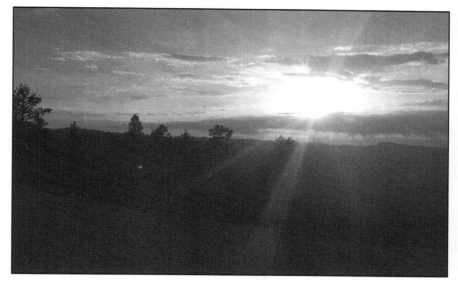

The sunrise at Grand Canyon.

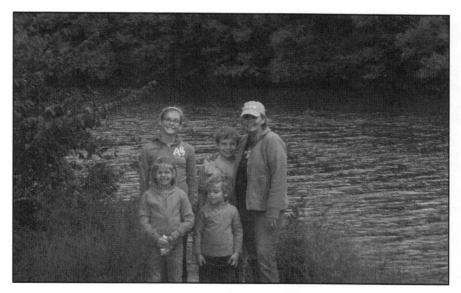

Enjoying some time in nature with the kids.

Laura Dahl

ful, but the shops and restaurants filled the space where we were. When we left, Joe knew about the creek running along the road we had followed back toward the Grand Canyon. The kids were begging to stop and we finally found a small parking area that had a path down to the creek. Well, that was it! We could have completely skipped Sedona and stayed at the creek all day. We all found so much peace and beauty there. It was a blessing for us all.

We went up into Utah and stopped first at Arches National Park and then Bryce Canyon and finally Zion National Park. All were incredible and I feel so blessed that I got to see them. I guess it was more than just seeing, it was experiencing them. At Arches, we went on a horseback trail and a Colorado River ride. Then we went on to Bryce Canyon National Park, which was unbelievably beautiful as well. At the top of the ridge (at about 8900 ft) there was a magnificent, almost 360 degree view out across the plain, filled with rock formations and bronze plaques with quotes framed inside a covered display. I thought this quote was particularly beautiful:

"I need solitude. I have come forth to this hill...to see the forms of the mountains on the horizon – to behold and commune with something grander than man."
- Henry David Thoreau Journal, August 14, 1854

Zion National Park was also impressive and maybe the most beautiful. We got to celebrate my parents' 45th wedding anniversary and had a lot of fun and a lot of great food. Unfortunately my mother passed out while we were visiting the park and Joe and I followed the ambulance to the hospital which was (in)conveniently located in St. George, Utah, about

35 miles away. Thankfully, it just turned out to be heat exhaustion and probably some dehydration. We got to leave the hospital a couple of hours later. Thankfully, Joe drove slower and a little closer to the yellow lines between the lanes on the way back. I think my constant praying helped too!

Speaking of constant praying, maybe you've noticed that one of the most difficult parts of living with cancer is dealing with the ups and downs. Yes, just a little difficult. And the crazy thing is that even though cancer is a physical illness, often with physical problems, it can be hard to know what's really going on. I have had quite a few doctor and nurse appointments where I went in feeling pretty good and came out on the verge of tears. What is that depressing saying? Nothing gold can last forever. I had another MRI and results weren't great. Not horrible but not good. Thank goodness God has been with me the whole time.

Caring Bridge
Written August 27, 2012 10:38am

Hello all - hope you've all had a wonderful summer - we sure did. After our trip out West (which I didn't forget about the pictures, I tried to post some but the files are too big - I'll try to work on that) we headed South to visit with family and had a fantastic time! Lots of sun, swimming, beach and just good fun.

In the meantime, I went out to Boston at the end of July just for a checkup and reload on my meds. Two days after we got back home from our trip South, I had a little "episode" (for lack of a better word) and got a quick trip to the ER. Nobody's really sure what happened but with my brain, it was likely treatment-related swelling so they put me on steroids for a few weeks and it's been fine. I'm just sorry the whole thing freaked the kids out. I am very thankful to my wonderful friends and neighbors for helping out so much!

Laura Dahl

I went back to Boston last Thursday and Friday for scans and a checkup. I wasn't really expecting the results to be great because of what happened. They showed that things are over all, stable in my brain – but that's only what the trial language says. In actuality, 2 of the three measurable tumors grew, but overall I am still below my baseline from May. The neuro-radiologist who did the initial report thinks that might be radiation injury rather than tumor growth. On the CT scan, something very light showed up on the lungs, but the report indicates that it's probably viral related. All in all, I guess it's not bad, but still, disappointing – growth is never a good word when it comes to cancer. I had put a lot of hope in this trial drug and it doesn't seem to be working as well as we thought it would. Don't get me wrong, the label "stable" is a very good thing and I wouldn't mind a bit if I could stay stable for a very long time. I guess we just have to wait and see what the next 8 week holds. If I start to experience any symptoms I'll be getting scanned again much sooner.

We also discussed another clinical trial that's a new chemo looking at Her2+ cancer brain mets. The good news is that I would probably be able to get on a trial much closer to home, either Chicago or Indianapolis. Bad news is that it's a traditional chemotherapy and comes with all the cr*p that goes along with that. I am experiencing almost no side effects on the drug I am on now and it's been so nice! But, I will do what I have to do. I know God has a plan for me and I'm totally on board with whatever that is, but I sure do hope for another 13 years. That's when I feel like my job, being a mother to 4 amazingly talented, beautiful children could technically be called finished. Aaron just started Kindergarten this year, and will graduate from High School in June of 2025. That's my date, my goal – as unrealistic as it may be. I have let God know about this plan, but also told Him that I understand that it's not my will to be done, but His. I trust He knows what He's doing with this life. Seeing Aaron graduate will be *a huge accomplishment, probably the biggest of my entire life and a great testament to God's mercy and love. But, every day is a miracle for me at this point and I am thankful for each one. I hope that I can make each day from now until my last, whenever that may be, a great testament to God's Love.*

God answers prayers and I am so glad you all are keeping me and my family in yours.

Peace,
Laura

Well, of course things didn't get better. One thing I have learned in receiving cancer treatment meds is that once they stop working, the cancer resumes its soulless trajectory. I was really upset learning the drug was not going to work for me. When Dr. Freedman first told me about it and its benefits, I had such high hopes. I thought this was it - I was going to go on this drug and be able to live a long time. It was going to work!

But apparently not...

Goodbye Boston, I'll miss you
Written October 21, 2012 12:58pm

Actually, I hope to be back. It's a cool city and I really want to take the kids there and see the wonderful sights, and maybe I'll remember how to navigate the T. For now though, I had to say goodbye. My results from the scans I had Thursday showed definite progression and that means the drug I was on clearly wasn't working. All the tumors they were measuring for the trial and the small, random ones spread around my brain they were watching, all grew over the last 8 weeks. Which sucks. I had a lot of hope in this drug to keep me stable for a long time. And I really liked my Doctor. And I loved staying with Bill and Betsy – I am so thankful to them and so thankful for getting to know them better!

So now what? I can't remember what plan that was, C...D? Whatever, we're moving on to the next one, hopefully anyway. There is another trial drug that my Dr. recommended and they have 2 study sites in Illinois - one in Harvey and one in Chicago. This clinical trial is the one I mentioned before that's a chemotherapy drug, but I will probably receive Herceptin as well. I am going to try to get an appointment ASAP and get started ASAP too.

I was accompanied this trip by my amazing, wonderful SIL Mandy (whose Aunt is Betsy) and we got to have some fun and got to eat some amazing food. She was with me in the doctor's office when I got the news and it was so comforting having her with me, though I'm sorry she suffered the news with me. With her loving heart, knowing at that time I needed to find some Peace, she suggested we find a church, and she did (love iphones!). A beautiful old church near Harvard called St. Paul's. And though I was still reeling a bit, I did find it there - I think God always comes to us like that and brings His Peace and Hope and Joy to those who need it at the very moment we need it most.

Today at church, the readings really brought me a lot of Peace too, especially the Responsorial Psalm, from number 33: "Our soul waits for the LORD, who is our help and shield. May your kindness, O LORD, be upon us who have put our hope in you.

Lord, let your mercy be on us, as we place our trust in you"

We have an absolutely gorgeous day today, which I am so thankful for – as I am thankful for them all.

Peace,
Laura

Harvey

Be joyful in hope, patient in affliction, faithful in prayer.
~ Romans 12:12

As I have progressed through this cancer journey, there have been many new experiences, some of them good, of course, but most have been difficult. In August 2012, after learning about the growing tumors, I started to experience headaches and then had a strange experience with a temporary loss of my language skills and a bad headache. Of course Steve was out of town (yet again!) and in Chicago, but luckily a couple of incredible friends, Marie and Patty (who happen to be sisters) were available. They rushed over and called 911 for me while Steve (probably) raced home. It must have been such a difficult ride for him. Thankfully I started to feel better once I got to the hospital and had gotten all my language back by the time he arrived. Really, I had started to feel much better while in the ambulance and once we

Laura Dahl

got to the ER I was ready to turn around and go back home. Steve showed up a little later and the doctor let us go. My wonderful neighbor Diane had snuck on to the ambulance and I didn't even know it until the next day when we talked about it!

So, moving onward, we went to Harvey, Illinois to talk about my next treatment, another clinical trial. This one sounded really interesting as it was chemotherapy with an acid peptide attached to it to help the drug cross the blood brain barrier. The hospital, Ingall's Memorial, turned out to be located in an interesting part of Chicago, but really easy for us to get to, taking about two hours from home. The people who worked there were very polite and friendly. I don't think there was a time we went that one of the employees didn't say hello, ask how things were going, if they could help, or if we needed anything. I noticed this trait on my first visit and it made a great first impression. The hospital itself was alright – old, but being refurbished - but the staff really made a huge impression. After being treated at one of the world's top hospitals (Dana Farber), it was so nice to go to a small community hospital that could help me with a new drug while treating others with a great kindness.

Next moves
Caring Bridge, Written October 30, 2012 9:48am

Whew, things have been a little crazy round here since I got back from Boston a little more than a week ago. I was feeling alright (well, disappointed) but by Tuesday morning I had started to get a pretty bad head ache and then other strange stuff with my brain started getting worse – difficulty communicating, and vision problems. Finally Steve took me to the hospital and they did another CT scan of my head which showed that the lesions had started to swell and were causing the symptoms. Got started on IV steroids and felt much better by midnight and by Wednesday morning had no side effects from the swelling, just really tired and a little fuzzy from the steroids and been about the same since then. I am to see Dr. Rowland tomorrow to hopefully wean down the steroids starting tomorrow.

In the mean time, I had been (and currently am) working on getting on the new clinical trial. Steve and I went up to the new hospital (which is not new at all, but about 100 years old but just as cute as can be and the people were super nice) and got the tour and I got 4 out of the 5 tests I needed to get done. I have to go back this Thursday for the final one and then should be able to start the new trial the following Thursday!

Hoping, hoping, hoping of course that this med will work! Should be easier to get up to Harvey, it's only a 2 hour car ride and should be a one day infusion. Days with scans will obviously take another day, but we'll cross the bridge as we get there.

Thanks all so much for continuing to pray. And special thanks to friends Patty and Marie who took care of the kids when I had to go to the hospital and for our wonderful meals we had the special treat of having. I may need to ask people for rides, still unsure when I will be allowed to drive again, but hopefully in the near term. I feel very much surrounded by love and concern – I love you all too!

Peace,
Laura

After a difficult start, the new treatment finally happened at Harvey on Nov 10, 2012. In early December I had the first scans for the new treatment and they were very good, showing "significant progress!" Perfect Christmas gift!

In the beginning, the drug was pretty manageable and I only

had to go to Harvey every three weeks. I still needed some injections for blood counts and bone strength, which were on different schedules, so Dr. Starr (the new doctor) let me get them at our house in Mahomet. Steve quickly learned how to give injections and it turned out that he has kind of a gift with giving shots and they hardly hurt!

By the end of January, the drug had started to bother me and I ended up losing all my hair. Again. For the third time. Winter 2013 was pretty rough. I also started to feel worse after each treatment and I slept through my time at the hospital and then most of the next day. But it was working – the scans were showing marked improvement. And so we continued. It was pretty much the same thing for the rest of the time I was on this trial. Of course, the weather improved finally, and we got to go to Florida in between treatments.

By the end of September though, questions started to arise about the drug's efficacy. There was some initial confusion and the radiologist who had been reading all my MRIs during the trial went on vacation, but when he returned and we got the results in October, they weren't good. The nurse (Toya – one of my best, friendliest nurses) and I talked on the phone and she explained the tumor had started to grow again. She made sure, though, that I knew it was still better than when I started the last November. I am so thankful for that trial and for the staff at Ingall's Memorial Hospital. On to the next phase, though.

While the end of the trial was going on, I had made appointments to see Dr. Rowland about what we could do locally at Carle. Traveling 20 minutes would be much better than 2 hours driving to Harvey or 3 hours by plane in Dana Farber's case. Karen and I had been looking at nearby trials because Carle didn't have one available. Karen found that the one in Chicago was actually using three drugs which had already been approved by the FDA and were available for all the public to use. When Dr, Rowland heard of the drugs, he was on board with going forward, but had a concern about my insurance paying for the newest chemotherapy part of the combo (Afinitor – the new one – Navelbine, and Herceptin) because I was not on the trial.

Well, I apparently have really good insurance (I knew this) because they said they'd pay for all the drugs. Thankfully, it seems to be working, although not spectacularly. While there is no improvement, it is working by holding the tumors stable. I'm good with that for now. The problems I'm having from the drugs aren't particularly fun or comfortable, but they are tolerable. We have been looking at other clinical trials, but there are very few available that I would qualify for (like two) and they would involve travel. Sigh. I'm hoping that, for the foreseeable future, my Afinitor combo keeps things steady.

Laura Dahl

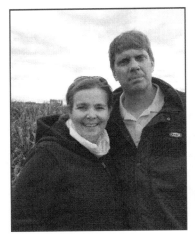

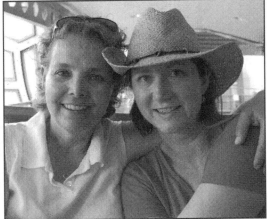

Field trip.

Love, support, and a great hat!
Thanks, Mandy!

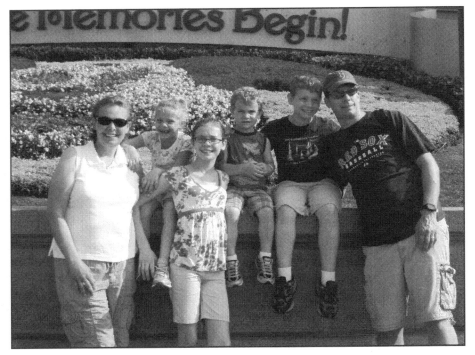

The Dahl family loves Disney!

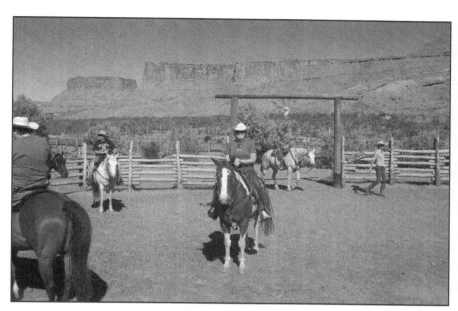

Horseback riding at Arches National Park.

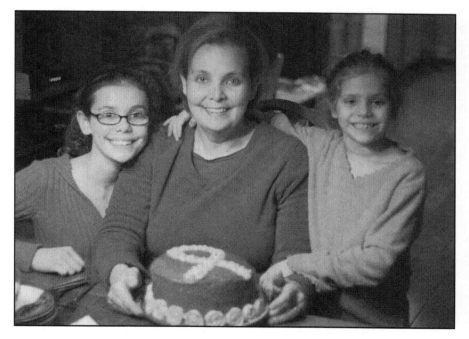

Rachel, Laura & Katherine with pink ribbon cake
3rd Cancerversary – Feb. 5, 2011

Laura Dahl

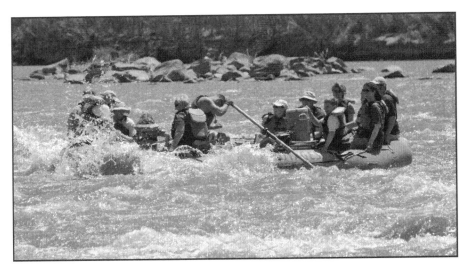

Colorado River rafting was fun!

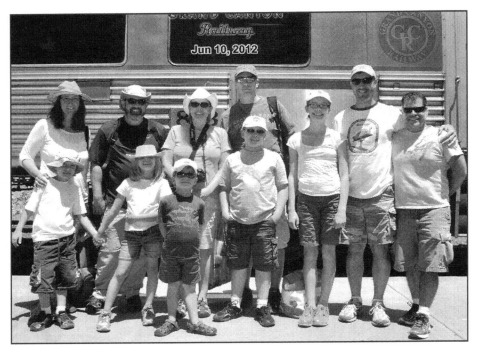

Traveling to the Grand Canyon.

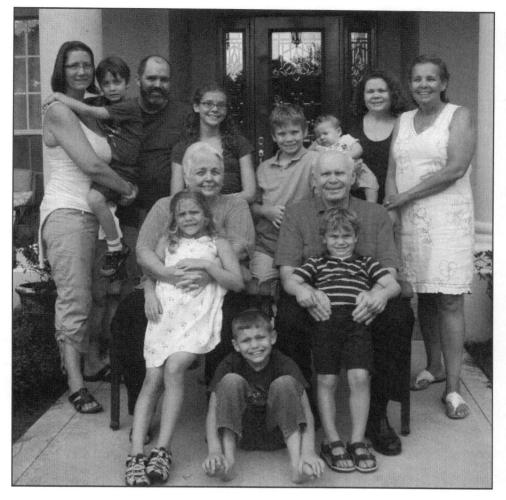

Precious times together as a family.

Laura Dahl

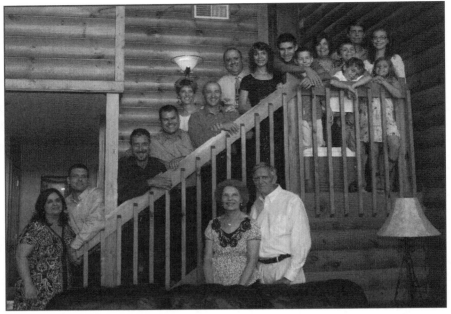

Dahl family gathering, 2013, Steve's parents' 50th anniversary.

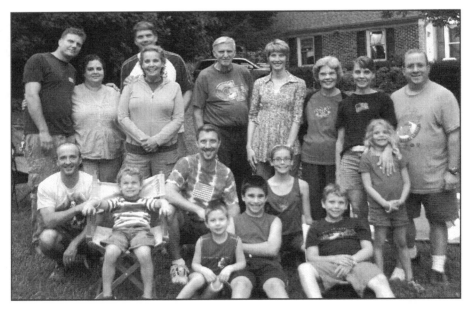

Now there's a good-looking family!

2009:
Disney just a few weeks
before the word
"cancer"came in to
our lives.

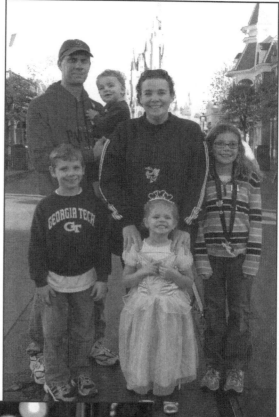

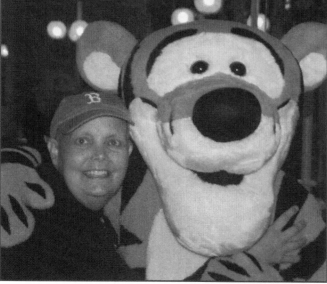

Like I said, our
family REALLY
loves our trips to
Disney!

Laura Dahl

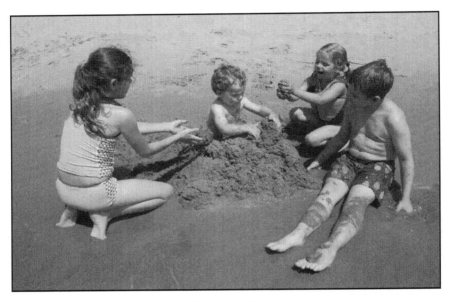

My angels in the sand, Summer 2009.

it's a Wonderful life

What a wonderful life I've had! I only wish I'd realized it sooner.
~ Coletterishikajain.com

God has blessed me in innumerable ways. I'm not sure when the thought started to really grow its roots in my conscious, but I have realized that my life is good. God has helped me understand that this life is in answer to a very specific prayer of mine. He has helped me understand how incredibly blessed I am. And He has let me truly see how wonderful each day is. I'd love to say that I thank Him each day for my life, with its warts and all, but I get distracted pretty easily. My brain is a little bit fried and it's a lot harder to stay focused now. Gosh, does that sound like a bunch of excuses or what? See, that proves how human this process is.

I named this last chapter after my very favorite movie because that's how I feel about my life too. Has it been perfect?

Laura Dahl

No, far from it! But, in spite of that, I have been immensely blessed in so many ways and I hope I can tell people about it. That's really what I wanted to do with this book. I want people to understand how much good can come from the difficult, the impossible... and how amazing God is at all times.

A lot of people wonder about living with cancer and imagine how hard it must be, and they're right, it is. Dealing with chemo treatment, travel, doctor appointments, scans, tests, blood draws is unbelievably difficult sometimes. But there are so many good days stuck in there – there's a silver lining. Praise God, there's always a good thing about each day.

After reading through my Caring Bridge entries again, I realized how many good reports I had – how many wonderful trips we went on – how many happy times we've experienced. Now, clearly there's a lot more tough news than good, but that I included as much good as I did is a success in itself. I think at one point I realized that even though I had had many bad days to report in the first couple of years, there were over 700 good days! That's fantastic, right!? But it gets so much better. Now, after five-plus years, it's been over 1,800 amazing days! In living with stage 4 Cancer, many of the reports you receive are plastered with medical jargon that you happily can't understand. As I moved on with my treatment, I got to learn a lot more about this disease. Even though you might think you don't want to know any more about it, I have always felt better as I learned more because the more I knew, the more I could do to slow it down, and the more time I knew I'd have with my family (say another 3,200 days, at least?)!

One of the problematic things about stage 4 cancer is of course that you really don't know how much time you've got left on this planet. Many of you will say, well none of us knows how much time we've got. And yes that's true, but it's much easier to imagine your 80's and 90's when you don't have this awful diagnosis on your back. Stage 4 Cancer notoriously cuts life considerably shorter – more reason to enjoy every day and be thankful!

Though 2013 turned out to be less than optimal, with many down spots to go overcome, we made it! The first part of the year was especially difficult for me for several reasons. The first was that winter had turned ugly and miserable for me, an avowed anti-winter citizen. When combined with a difficult treatment, travel two hours to South Chicago every three weeks, and a husband who had to travel every week for his current project to Springfield, MO, times were rough. My prayer life was even suffering. Thankfully God doesn't give up when things get tough. I made it through that winter and as soon as Spring came, my outward appreciation of all life came back. Not that it was all gone, just pretty difficult to see. We got to celebrate Steve's parents' 50th wedding anniversary that July. All of Steve's family met at Gatlinburg, TN and we spent three days catching up, going to the tourist traps, playing games, and just enjoying all being together. Then we went down to stay with my parents in Jacksonville, FL – a trip I have looked forward to almost every year for many years. Katherine once asked me if we would ever get a vacation home (we had been watching HGTV) and I told her "we already do! Grandma and Grandpa's house in Florida!" And she vociferously agreed (laughing and yelling her agreement)!

Even though 2013 was one of the toughest years, it clearly wasn't without its fun. After I met my mother's writing friend in Jacksonville, we hit a stride! I can't tell everyone how thankful I am for Susan. She is an amazing person, full of faith, and has made this book possible. When I first spoke to her in Florida that summer, I knew she was special and I looked very forward to her help. But not only was she going to do that, she put us in touch with an organization helping women get to Orlando to have some crucial R&R. After I returned to Illinois and while we were writing, she told me about "Memories of Love" in Jacksonville, and she put me in touch with them. With some difficulty (because our fall schedule had been crazy), I got to talk to them and arrange a trip to Universal, Sea Word and Disney in November for a week. Their generosity and help was so wonderful – we will thank them and remember them always.

By the way, my beautiful and loving Aunt Karen passed away in 2012. She always made me feel special and loved. Susan reminds me of her – a fantastic woman who knows how to keep running up with life and that there's lots more ahead both for herself and lots of others, too!

The trip to Orlando was fantastic and a major blessing (on top of that, after we left Illinois, it snowed). It was in the 60's and 70's in Orlando. Thank you Jesus for that major blessing – I appreciate it! We got our free tickets for Universal Orlando, Islands of Adventure, and Sea World from Memories of Love and then went to Disney for two days. It was so quick, but so much fun and I knew God was looking out for us too – a young guy and his girlfriend came up to me and asked to pray for me that second day and they did! What a beautiful gift from God!

I have always felt that my family is awesome and that they have been and always will be the greatest blessing from God. Writing this book has only strengthened this feeling and my great love for them. I've also gotten to seriously contemplate how blessed I am. Clearly, my husband and children are God's greatest gifts to me and although things don't always go the best, they are each sublime. I can't imagine life without them. God knows this too. At a Cursillo group meeting in 2004, I mentioned a prayer to my groupies that had recently come to me. When appreciating my life and my family in particular, I prayed to God this: *"God, if anything bad, I mean really bad, is going to happen in my life, let it be to me. Let this bad thing happen to me, not my family."* He was listening.

My children have been so amazing to me. I realize that's not saying a whole lot because most parents think the same way. But I guess I especially see them as gifts from God – their light shines continuously and I know it will never stop. They are my heart.

Each morning before they go to school, my children and I stand in a close circle and say this prayer: *"Dear Jesus – Thank you for this day and for all that we have. Continue to bless us and keep us safe. Help us to love and serve you always. Amen."*

I'm so thankful for my children.

Rachel is our 16-year-old and is playing her part as the oldest and most responsible so incredibly well. Actually, she is really amazing and, since she's been part of this planet, talented in so many different things. Ever since she was born, I have had an exceptional opinion of her, not that I'm biased of her incredibleness or anything. Now, that's not saying we've been without arguments throughout the years. It seems like it might be impossible for teenage daughters and their moms to get along all the time, but many times Rachel and I are fantastic together! She is highly intelligent and loves books, as I do! And she knows how to cook – pretty darn well too! Currently she is riding horses for a hobby (but gets to play on them riding in the English style). She's also gotten into some things in high school like Drama and Scholastic Bowl, and she's already starting to think about college and what she might want to do there - this doesn't seem quite possible to me and I'm very glad we've still got a couple years left to get it going.

Rachel has her own room with a queen-size bed. She moved in there quite a while ago and we allowed her to do that with the single exception that when somebody comes to stay, they get that room. Rachel is immaculate about her room and everything else. We don't have to worry about it being neat when company comes.

Looking back, one of my favorite memories of Rachel is when she started piano lessons at about 8 years old. She liked it at first but after a few years, she decided she didn't want to do it anymore. We talked about it and I told her she had to keep playing. She agreed, but after a few more weeks, she started complaining. "I hate this!" she'd say. "I want to quit!" Every time she had a lesson, I got an earful. I just kept telling her, "Rachel, I love you. We're going to do this and we're going to see this through." She had the same piano teacher all along, which was a saving grace because she loved her and she came to the house. Unfortunately, things changed as things have a way of doing – her piano teacher got married and moved, but by then, Rachel was in 8th grade and had started to enjoy playing the piano. She is good. I'm not just saying that because she's my daughter. She's good. Some time during the past year, she's started to play Mozart and Beethoven and Chopin and she really loves it. She actually told me thank you for keeping on her and not letting her quit, and now she can do this. She plays so beautifully – it is a real talent. I once told her that someday she'd thank me and now she has. In fact, now when I listen to my daughter play beautiful music, I thank her.

Or second child is **Ben**, our incredible genius. Well, his brain is exceptional and because of it, he's had a lot of trouble with school – not skipping, but intensely ahead anyway, and just managing not to fall asleep each day. Since he was in 1st grade, we've known there was something special about his intelligence. I told you that Rachel is smart, but Ben's intellect goes beyond any of the other children, but his common sense can't even compare to Rachel's. Like Einstein, Ben's ability to handle life stuff is sometimes a challenge. He is brilliant, but can barely make sure his teeth are brushed every day and his work is done on time. Sometimes he's so bored with the homework, he just puts it down somewhere and misplaces it. Luckily, Ben has been able to keep up and maintain his A's for the school work he's handed in. Unfortunately, almost all the work he's had to do is far below his abilities and he's been bored to tears. Finally in 6th grade we were able to get him moved up at least in math. I called the principal and just wanted him to look at Ben's ISAT state scores and let me know what he thought. Illinois hands out "MAP" testing frequently to show how the students are doing in each grade, past elementary. One afternoon Ben came home and was joking with Rachel about their MAP Scores and we were all in for a shock when he just mentioned them. Rachel was in 8th grade and in Algebra 1, Ben in 6th grade and in 6th grade honors. His test scan that spring was 237. Rachel's was 224. Ben's principal also looked up his 5th grade scores and the test came back that he had a perfect score on the math (this very rarely happens). Of course, it was obvious to me already. Even though he was only in 6th grade, the 8th grade Algebra 1 math teacher (also a

Laura Dahl

friend from church) thought he could do it too. In 7th grade, Ben began Algebra 1 and hasn't looked back since. He had no problems skipping three grades in math his 7th grade year and this year has Honors Geometry, a sophomore high school class. He got an A+ last year and is getting an A+ right now in Geometry. Unfortunately, there are not many other classes he could move forward on, but we'll be having meetings with the high school staff soon before he begins at the high school in the fall. The last time I checked, he told us he was going to MIT. I'm good with that, I think – isn't that too far away?

At 13, Ben's got some very close friends and is well-liked. Everybody knows he's smart, and he's the most easygoing of all of us. Ben does what I ask him to do right away, unless he's reading... then we call him the absent minded professor. He gets this from my dad. If he's reading, forget about talking to him. You have to go up to him and say, "Hey Ben," to get his attention. His newest thing is an obsession with a four-inch screen that he shares with some close friends. They can play Minecraft games for hours – some of his friends came over on a Saturday at 10 a.m. and played all day until 8 p.m. I just let them, but their moms and I joke we might have to do an intervention for their "addiction."

Miss **Katherine**, my little love. Steve and I decided we were ready for another child when Ben finally figured out how to sleep at about four (from the time he was 3 months old when he caught a virus, Respiratory Syncytial Virus (RSV), Ben had trouble sleeping). Anyway, I was ready for another child and boy, were we blessed with Katherine. She is just so incredibly bright and loving.

When she was born, Steve and I actually didn't know if she was a boy or girl. The doctor had pulled the baby down to relieve the fluid from the breathing right after she was born and, as you probably figured out, this made it quite difficult to see the baby. Once we heard the doctor say the baby was fine, we both asked at the same time if it was a boy or girl. "Oh, sorry – it's a girl!"

And what a girl! She was amazingly beautiful! So small, too – although the hospital said she was 8 pounds, she looked smaller (much smaller than Rachel at 8'10 and Ben at 9'2). She also was just the sweetest baby we'd ever seen. She hardly cried or made any kind of grouchy noise.

Now, in 3rd grade, she is still a special, friendly, smiling treat. Sometimes a bit smart-alecky, but almost always she has a smile on her face. The openness of her love is one of her biggest attributes and I pray God keeps her loving of others very special.

One of my favorite memories of Katherine was when her little brother, Aaron, was born. She was two years old and Steve brought all three of the kids to my hospital room. She, being the smallest, was trying to push in. "I want to hold he," she kept saying. When she finally got to hold him, her eyes lit up and sparkled with love.

Katherine does very well in school and is always ahead in reading and spelling. She loves art, especially drawing, and creates spectacular pictures in pencil, marker and/or crayon, and then she usually ends up giving them to me with so much love. I will always cherish them. My favorite thing about Katherine is the openness of her love. She is not shy at all to show how she feels.

Our little surprise, **Aaron**, has kept us constantly on our toes! After we had Katherine, both Steve and I agreed we were good when it came to children. Hah! I mentioned that thing about giving God a good laugh by telling Him your plans, right? (That

Laura Dahl

pretty much goes with the cancer thing, too). I learned I was pregnant with Aaron in the fall of 2006, and to be quite honest, I wasn't the most excited. Since he was going to be number four, I mentioned to God that I might be finished in this role. Again, remember what I said before about making God laugh! My time pregnant with Aaron flew by and since I had all the other kids by induction using the drug called oxyeitocin, I just decided to go ahead and make plans with our doctor for the same. If for some reason he came earlier, well that'd be okay with us! Of course he didn't come early (as none of the others had) and on July 19, 2007 he came at quite a stroll - I hardly felt any contractions until that night and then all of a sudden, he was there! Amazing and wonderful, intelligent and beautiful! He was to complete the symphony that is our family. I knew he was the last, but it has been so worth having him with us.

His childhood so far has been the most difficult of all of the children because of the cancer. Remember, when I was first diagnosed with Cancer, I was only 38 and he was 19 months old. In a lot of ways I tried to keep focused on him in particular so that he could remember me after I passed away. Now that he's 6, working on 7, I think that at least he's got a much better chance of remembering me. We have been such close partners since that first treatment. I have put an effort into helping him learn specific things, like faith and love. As with most last born kids, though, he's got quite a lot to prove and he lets us hear about it! He likes his own way and seems to be 6 going on 36 with the amount of stuff coming out of that mouth. We're also learning how smart he is. Already in 1st grade, he is one of the best math students and reads incredibly well. Unfortunately, he also challenges us all on, well, just about everything. I'm at least thankful that he is a huge snuggler and. really, I get the majority of that love.

Aaron loves to play chess and is highly competitive. In the beginning, when I was playing with this smart little four year-old, I'd show him where he made a mistake and let him take it back. That no longer happens. He's a good chess player. He loves cards, too, and scrabble – all board games. He likes to play with my parents and, especially with Rachel – hardly anybody can beat her at Risk and she used to love Monopoly. Aaron can play that game and win. Unfortunately, he can be a bad loser – he wants to go first and he wants to be in charge, but he's gotten better lately. Last summer, Joe taught the kids to play poker with a bunch of chips. They love to play games.

The children have been an enormous blessing from heaven and without them, my life would be completely missing their love, their life, and their shine – a life I am incredibly grateful God chose differently for me. God dwelling in me is the essence of His Grace in me, in my heart and soul. I pray almost daily for God to endow them with His Spirit always and help them live safely at peace and with happiness. My children are the most brilliant lights in my life and they shine for me.

Steve. *My Rock. My Love.* He is the kind of man that women hope for – solid, committed, loving. I have him. And no, you can't. We didn't always have the greatest relationship through college, but I know that marrying Steve was the pinnacle of my life – the best thing I ever did. He completed me. (Yeah, I know that's from the movie, Jerry Maguire) but he did and he is one of the most dedicated and committed people I have ever known. Plus, he loves me! I was, and always will be, an incredibly lucky wife. I am so proud and honored to be his wife and I pray every-day for us to be together as long as possible.

The children know how important our faith is to Steve and me. He feels very strongly about making sure we go to worship and religious education. I talk about it a lot easier than he does – but I know his feelings. He backs me up. Unless you're really sick, you're going to church. We don't want to be the parents who shoved it down their throats, but we pray in the morning, we pray at dinner and we pray at bedtime. All I want is for them to have a love of God in their life. I believe Christianity is the way to do that. It's important to us to make sure that God is a huge part of their lives. He needs to be central in their lives – if they can get out of college and marry someone who believes in God, then we've been successful.

Rachel went to a Catholic work camp we had signed her up for when she was in 8th grade. It was a great opportunity for her to start to build appreciation for what God has done in our lives. We paid the money – attended the meetings – raised the money – and she was supposed to go in June. She went to a meeting in April or May and came home and said she wasn't going. Steve and I looked at her and said, "Yes you are." She was adamant about not going. Something had turned her off and she wanted nothing to do with it. We forced her to go and she came home and said, "That was one of the best things I've ever done, Mom." I was so happy that I just about hit the floor. She said she couldn't wait for next year. She went again this past spring and is ready and raring to go again. This year, Ben is going, too. We are together in God.

Friends are another of God's great blessings. If someone had told me back in 2001 that I would love living in dry, flat, occasionally completely brown, cold Illinois, I would have fallen down laughing, or possibly crying. Steve and I discussed the move after he accepted the job from Kraft. I expected to live up here two years, max. I could handle that, right? I wouldn't need too many friends, I had my family. Amazing how little I knew back then and how few friends I had. Thank you God for the great gift of many, many people I now call friends. Please continue to bless them and keep them safe, happy and healthy!

My friends have been incredible partners in my fight. They have been with me since day one and I know they will never stop fighting my disease with me. They have invested greatly in me and I am incredibly in their debt. I love you all.

My rules for a happy, fulfilled life:

1. Have a strong faith. God is your number one ally and friend in life – He is Love! Let Him live in you, guide you and hold you. Live in this order: God, family, friends, world.

2. Spread the Love. Be an instrument of God's Peace, beginning with your family. And don't forget to smile.

3. Keep close to your family and friends. Their importance won't be fully felt until they are needed most. And choose the right ones – good heart, loyal, follower of Christ.

> *"Surround yourself only with people who are going to lift you higher." ~ Oprah*

There are many things I still need to do in this life (besides finishing this book) and one of the most important to me is helping with the hunger problem. I have helped previously in a very small way, but I feel pulled to work more and help our community. I'm of the opinion that there currently shouldn't be anyone in my town of 7000 who needs to wait in line for some others to fill their basket. We have enough. We have more than enough. It's my hope that I can interest enough people (this shouldn't be a problem, because I have some awesomely caring friends) to eradicate hunger in Mahomet. After that's completed, we'll have to go wider and wider. In my lifetime, it sure would be incredible to help so many people come out from the pain of hunger. Please pray for me to have the time and energy to do this. I'll need all that I can get!

"Those who are wise will shine like the brightness of the heavens, and those who lead many to righteousness, like the stars forever and ever." - Daniel 12:3 (NIV)

My favorite prayer that I try to say every morning:

Mother Teresa and the Missionaries of Charity
Daily Morning Prayer (mine too!):

"Dear Jesus, Help me to spread thy fragrance everywhere I go. Flood my soul with thy Spirit and Love. Penetrate and possess me so utterly that every soul I come into contact with will feel thy presence in my soul. Let them look up and see no longer me, but only you. Stay with me and then I shall begin to shine as you shine, so to shine as to be a light for others."

My Work for Jesus

So since Cursillo I have felt a great call from God asking me to help Him spread His Word, His Love. He hasn't directly spoken to me, but I have heard Him and felt Him. I think I said before that I knew He needed me to help spread His Love. I started easy by helping at Cursillo during almost every weekend they had, and I usually helped in the Kitchen and the prayer chapel. I knew I was working for Jesus and helping spread His message and most importantly, His Love. I prayed that the people I was serving through the weekend had an experience like I had. Well, I don't think that happened, but I know that many had great, spiritually uplifting experiences that affect them still today.

Even though my cancer has made it much more difficult to help at Cursillo weekends, I still try to stay involved as much as I can. I have listened to Christian radio and heard about charities needing specific things collected and mentioned these at church. And I hear about world wide problems and try to help there too. I also have been looking for things I can do for our local church, Our Lady of the Lake, and have recently been inspired by a book given to me by Mandy, entitled "7, An Experimental Mutiny Against Excess."

I made a list of projects I have worked on over the last 10 years, and as I listed them, boy, did I get a reminder of the work that still needs to be done!

At Our Lady of the Lake:
- Teaching Religious Education – grades Kindergarten, 2nd Grade, 3rd Grade, 5th Grade.
- Eucharistic Minister
- Women's Club
- Annual Food Collections at Thanksgiving
- Decorating for Holidays Collections for other charities
- Additional collections - shoes for orphans, local food

drives, money to Africa (by myself and with church friends – Sandee Aune), Shoes for Orphan Soles

Restoration Urban Ministries
- Serving Restoration Urban Ministries (RUM) Cursillo candidates
- Serve on Teams, including Rectora
- Collecting food, preparing dinners
- Clothing and grocery donations
- Financial Donations

Cursillo
- Served on 4 teams
- Prepared cooked items needed for weekends
- Served in the kitchen, Candidate's Chapel, Palanca Chapel, Registration, attending weekend events, Ultreyas

These are my primary philanthropic focuses and I love them all so much. I hope there is a day soon that I can go back to some! Of course, I have also focused on raising money for all of them too. After reading "7" and hearing from Mnsr. Ramer about acting on God's calling – we need to put our calls into actual physical work. And there's a lot to be done! This is the year I want to really start to focus on physically getting people some help, starting with those suffering from hunger and homelessness. It is my prayer that this book will be part of my ministry for Jesus.

Favorite Quotes

"You and I have been created for greater things. We have not been created to just pass through this life without aim. And that greater aim is to love and be loved. You are God's good news; you are God's love in action…each time people come into contact with us, they must become different and better people for having met us. We must radiate God's love."

~Mother Teresa

"Beloved, let us love one another, because love is of God; everyone who loves is begotten by God and knows God…No one has ever seen God. Yet if we love one another, God remains in us and His love is brought to perfection in us."

~1 John 4: 7-12

"We serve God by serving others. The world defines greatness in terms of power, possessions, prestige and position. If you can demand service from others, you've arrived. In our self-serving culture with its me-first mentality, acting like a servant is not a popular concept. Jesus, however, measured greatness in terms if service, not status. God determines your greatness by how many people you serve, not how many people serve you."

~Rick Warren

"Everybody can be great because anyone can serve. You don't have to have a college degree to serve. You don't have to make your subject and verb agree to serve. You only need a heart full of grace. A soul generated by love."

~Martin Luther King, Jr.

"Because of the tender mercies of my God by which the rising sun will come to me from heaven – to shine on my darkness and in what feels like the shadow of death to me – I will find

Laura Dahl

Peace."

~ Proverbs 31 Ministries (re-arranged from Bible quote)

Favorite Reads - Faithful

A Revolution of Love – The Meaning of Mother Teresa
David Scott

The Language of Love
Francis Collins

Where There is Love, There is God
Mother Teresa

Crossing the Threshfield of Hope
Pope John Paul II

Civilization of Love
Carle Anderson

The Reason for God
Tim Keller

Captivating
John and Stasi Elderidge

7: An Experimental Mutiny Against Excess
Jen Hatmaker

The Lamb's Supper
Scott Hahn

The Purpose Driven Life
Rick Warren

Mere Christianity
C.S. Lewis

Recipes for my family and friends

Dorie Greenspan: Baking, From My House to Yours

Tall and Creamy Cheesecake
http://www.seriouseats.com/recipes/2008/04/
creamy-cream-cheese-cheesecake-for-passover-recipe.html
Chocolate Biscotti
http://www.browneyedbaker.com/2008/09/15/
chocolate-biscotti/
World Peace Cookies
http://food52.com/blog/9299-pierre-herme-dorie-
greenspan-s-world-peace-cookies
Crème Brulee
http://someneedfulthings.blogspot.com/2011/08/
baking-with-dorie-creme-brulee.html

Laura Dahl

Sweet Potato Mallow
http://www.justapinch.com/recipes/side/potatoes/
sweet-potato-mallow.html

Millionaire Salad
http://www.foodily.com/r/PF1PMvBzTg-
millionaire-salad-by-cooking-light

Maple Bourbon Pecan Pie
http://www.marthastewart.com/333110/
maple-bourbon-pecan-pie

Christmas

Standing Rib Roast
http://www.marthastewart.com/343283/prime-rib

Yorkshire Pudding
http://www.marthastewart.com/339841/yorkshire-pudding

Red Velvet Cake
http://community.tasteofhome.com/community_forums/
f/30/p/12130/504073.aspx

Other Loved Recipes

Muffaletta Olive Salad
http://www.nolacuisine.com/2005/07/17/
muffuletta-sandwich-recipe/

Chicken Fricassee with Orzo – Cooking Light April 2000
http://www.myrecipes.com/recipe/
chicken-fricassee-with-orzo-10000000222416

Panera Broccoli Cheese Soup – Recipe Zarr
http://www.food.com/recipe/copycat-olive-garden-
minestrone-soup-by-todd-wilbur-77585

Creamy Lentil Soup – Cooking Light 2000
http://www.myrecipes.com/recipe/
creamy-lentil-soup-10000000665473

Copycat Olive Garden Soup – Todd Wilber
http://www.food.com/recipe/copycat-olive-garden-
minestrone-soup-by-todd-wilbur-77585

Poached Pear and Raspberry Trifle – Food Network
http://www.foodnetwork.com/recipes/emeril-lagasse/
poached-pear-and-raspberry-trifle-recipe.html

One Bowl Chocolate Cake – Martha Stewart
http://www.marthastewart.com/340315/
one-bowl-chocolate-cake

New York Crumb Cake – Martha Stewart
http://www.marthastewart.com/355763/
new-york-crumb-cake

Grandmother Paula's Sour Cream Pound Cake – Paula Dean
http://www.foodnetwork.com/recipes/paula-deen/
grandmother-pauls-sour-cream-pound-cake-recipe.print.html

Laura Dahl

Golden Mable Pumpkin Pie

http://www.marthastewart.com/314105/
maple-pumpkin-pie-with-leaf-lattice

Martha Stewart: Martha Stewart Baking Handbook

Banana Nut Bread

http://www.marthastewart.com/312772/banana-bread

Gingerbread Men

http://www.marthastewart.com/315628/
gingerbread-snowflakes

One Bowl Chocolate Cake

http://www.marthastewart.com/340315/
one-bowl-chocolate-cake

Pate Brisee

http://www.marthastewart.com/343815/pate-brisee

Thanksgiving

Roasted Turkey, brined

http://www.foodnetwork.com/recipes/alton-brown/
good-eats-roast-turkey-recipe.html

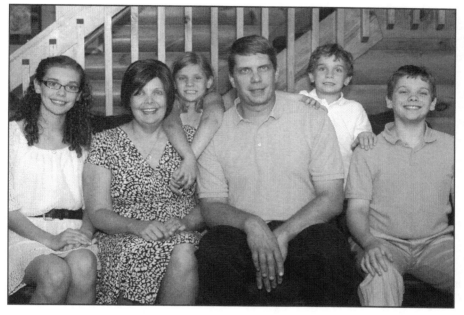

There's nothing as sweet as family time.

The Dahls - Summer 2013
in Gatlinburg, Tennessee at Grandma and Grandpa Dahl's
50th wedding anniversary celebration.

Laura Dahl

To order additional copies
of this book, please visit
http://www.amazon.com.